DEPRESSION
IN THE ELDERLY

DEPRESSION
IN THE ELDERLY

Conceptual Issues and
Psychotherapeutic Intervention

by
Walter S. Weinstein
Memphis State University

and
Prabha Khanna
Memphis State University

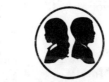

Philosophical Library
New York

Library of Congress Cataloging-in-Publication Data

Weinstein, Walter S.
  Depression in the elderly.

  Bibliography: p.
  Includes index.
  1. Geriatric psychiatry. 2. Depression,
Mental. I. Khanna, Prabha. II. Title.
  [DNLM: 1. Depression—in old age. 2. Psychotherapy—
in old age. 3. Psychotherapy, Group—in old age.
WM 171 W424d]
RC451.4.A5W428   1986   618.97'68527   85-16947
  ISBN 8022-2491-1

To
Our spouses, parents, and
grandparents

CONTENTS

Part Two
Psychotherapy Strategies

PART ONE

GENERAL CONSIDERATIONS

CHAPTER I

INTRODUCTION

The psychological problems of the elderly and the usefulness of psychotherapeutic interventions specifically geared towards them have received increased attention in the literature since the comprehensive review by Rechtschaffen (1959). This represented one of the first major attempts to document the special characteristics and modifications of psychotherapy which could most adequately address the psychological problems of the aged. It also served to crystallize issues surrounding the use of psychotherapy with the elderly and delineate more clearly its parameters.

3

Recently, several reviews have summarized the state of the art of psychotherapy with the elderly (Blank, 1974; Brink, 1979; Butler, 1975; Karpf, 1977; Knight, 1979; Peck, 1966; Sparacino, 1979; Willner, 1978). These reviews have generally supported Rechtschaffen (1959) in endorsing the usefulness of psychotherapeutic interventions with the elderly, while lamenting the continued lack of systematic evaluations of both therapy process and outcome. Based on available research, these reviewers were cautiously optimistic, suggesting that psychotherapy could alter the course of emotional problems by improving the ability of the aged person to adjust to change and manage the crises of later life.

Numerous authors (Brink, 1979; Butler, 1975; Kastenbaum, 1978; Verwoerdt, 1976) have documented data showing that the elderly are disproportionately subject to emotional as well as physical problems, and that, as a clinical entity, they are perhaps least likely to receive appropriate and adequate psychological treatment. A general consensus exists among many authors that depression represents the most pervasive manifestation of psychopathology exhibited by the elderly (Epstein, 1976; Gerner, 1979; Gottesman, Quarterman & Cohn, 1973; Karpf, 1977). As a prelude to a review of the utility of psychotherapy with depressed older persons, this book will briefly entertain several hypotheses regarding the connections between aging and depression. Changes in status, personality and cognition that come with age will be discussed in relation to the question of whether or not depression is a normal coping response in late life. A related issue to be discussed concerns the qualitative similarity of depression across the life span, i.e., how if it all, late life depressions differ from earlier depressions. Answers to these questions would be of obvious value in identification, diagnosis and selection of at-risk populations for purposes of prevention and treatment.

As discussed here, depression may be seen as a global and heterogeneous construct embracing a variety of symptoms, behaviors and possible causes (Akiskal, 1978; Akiskal & McKinney, 1975; Arieti, 1978). Problems encountered in psychotherapy with depressed elderly persons are compounded because the sequelae of depression are often inextricably intertwined and may be expressed both psychologically and physically. Thus, many physical symptoms and complaints in the elderly may actually mask the presence of a more basic underlying, depressive illness (Eisdorfer & Cohen, 1978; Gerner, 1979; Saltzman & Shader, 1978a). Prompt diagnosis and effective treatment of depression in the elderly are imperative in light of the compelling evidence showing that suicide rates peak in late life (Weiss, 1974) and that suicide attempts of the elderly are more likely to be successful.

Despite the problems of etiology and diagnosis of depression in the elderly, one should not conclude that psychotherapeutic treatment of depression is ruled out for this group. Because this issue has been a source of ongoing debate, this book will first address the question of whether in fact such therapy is actually possible or beneficial. Although the main focus will be upon verbal psychotherapy, this treatment is not universally preferred due to widespread reliance on pharmacology. Nevertheless, chemotherapy alone does not always constitute the most efficacious treatment. A proper perspective must be maintained in the use of antidepressant medications with the elderly (Fann, 1976; Fann & Wheless, 1975; Friedel, 1980; Salzman & Shader, 1978; Schmidt, 1974). In order to explore the relative merits of psychotherapy interventions in depressed elderly persons, both the advantages as well as some of the disadvantages and problems associated with drug treatment will be presented. Following the discussion of those issues, this book will document the use and relative effectiveness of various forms of individual and group psychotherapy as they apply to the treatment of depressed elderly persons. Adaptations and modifications of traditional, insight-oriented dynamic therapy will be discussed, as well as the subsequent move towards supportive therapies of briefer duration, the problem-solving, coping-skills training approach, and recent cognitive-behavioral strategies (Brink, 1979; Cath, 1972; Goldfarb, 1974; Kastenbaum, 1978; Sparacino, 1979). The relative advantages of group therapy will be explored and, in this context, the viability of the life review technique as a facilitator of insight and crisis resolution will be examined.

Scope and Magnitude of Depression in the Elderly

Depression is considered by many to be the most common emotional problem exhibited by the elderly (Butler & Lewis, 1973; Eisdorfer & Cohen, 1978). Others have noted that historically depression has been considered a concomitant of the aging process (Epstein, 1976; Grigorian, 1970). Pfeiffer and Busse (1973) indicated that affective disorders are by far the most frequently encountered form of psychopathology in the elderly, regardless of whether community-based outpatient or hospitalized populations are considered. These authors suggested that up to one-half of all psychiatric admissions of elderly people involve a diagnosis of some affective disorder.

Studies of geriatric outpatients have also indicated that about half appear to manifest depressions (Charatan, 1975; Roth, 1955). Dovenmuehle, Reckless & Newman (1970) found that about 30 percent of a general community population over sixty years of age exhibited depressive symptomatology. Another estimate of the prevalence of depression in an English community (Pitt, 1974) found some affective disturbance in 26 percent of those over age sixty-five. Feigenbaum (1970) reported that 52 percent of the diagnoses in one geriatric psychiatric outpatient clinic were for affective disorders, and that psychotic and neurotic depressions accounted for almost 95 percent of these.

Karpf (1977) noted that depression is a "singularly prevalent" disorder among the aged, and cited a survey by Busse, Barnes, Silverman, Thaler & Frost (1955), which found strong evidence of clinical depression in almost half of their sample of persons over age sixty who were unable to work and who were being treated for physical disorders on an outpatient basis. This same study suggested that almost as many depressive reactions were detected in retired individuals who were economically secure and in good physical health. Brink (1979) agreed that depression was the most typical psychiatric problem in old age, and that it constituted a majority of clinical cases. In terms of proportion of cases, the general finding repeatedly has been that the incidence of depression rises with advancing age (Levitt & Lubin, 1975; Scott & Gaitz, 1975; Swab, Holzer & Warheit, 1973).

Prevalence of depression varies from the less severe neurotic-reactive to the more severe psychotic-endogenous dichotomy (Spicer, Hare & Slater, 1973). Generally, neurotic depressions tend to peak for both sexes in the third decade and decline thereafter while psychotic depressions peak at about age sixty for males and about age fifty for females (Gerner, 1979). Gurland (1976) observed a higher incidence of depression in women than in men prior to age forty-five and a tendency for this trend to equalize and then reverse beyond age sixty-five.

However, Gurland (1976) has pointed out that methodological considerations and measurement difficulties cloud interpretations of the relationship between age, frequency and type of depression. Gurland (1976) argued that differences in age-related prevalence rates are often seen, depending upon whether clinical diagnoses of depressions or age patterns of depressive symptoms are reported. Thus, Gurland (1976) concluded that depressive disorders as diagnosed by psychiatrists are most frequent between the ages of twenty-five and sixty-five with a decline after age forty; but in studies where symptoms are analyzed, those over sixty-five have the greatest rates of depression.

Jarvik (1976) has also discussed nosological problems, which have resulted in a somewhat unclear picture of the prevalence of depression among the elderly. Jarvik (1976) agreed however, that persons age sixty-five and over, as a group, display the highest overall rates of depressive symptomatology. Blumenthal (1975) contended that these results may in fact be a consequence of the measuring devices used to assess the presence of depressive symptoms. Because many of the items of self-report scales used in these studies refer to physical or vegetative signs associated with depression, it is possible that high scores represent actual somatic complaints and not true depression. Thus, it has been suggested that inclusion of such items on a depression scale may result in spuriously high depression ratings when used with subjects who also manifest physical problems unrelated to depression.

Noting these problems and the potential for diagnostic confusion, Epstein (1976) discussed the danger of underestimating the pervasiveness of depression in the elderly and warned of harmful therapeutic consequences in cases where depression is misdiagnosed or left untreated to become progressively entrenched as a coping response. A vicious circle may begin with depression leading to apathy, isolation, poor nutrition and neglect of physical health, which then, in turn, fosters further depressive symptomatology.

CHAPTER II

IS PSYCHOTHERAPY BENEFICIAL?

According to Blank (1974) and Brink (1979) psychotherapeutic strategies imply the existence of a conscious mutual agreement between client and therapist in which a formal, disciplined method of helping the individual resolve mental distress is employed. Blank (1974) used this definition to differentiate psychotherapy from interventions which do not involve a formal, conscious agreement between client and therapist, such as reality therapy, activity therapy and milieu therapies. Brink (1979) described psychotherapy as a "process of interaction" which focuses on communication between client and therapist. He cautioned, however, that communication serves only as a vehicle for facilitating treatment and that undue emphasis should not be placed on the quality of the verbal skills of the elderly person. Brink (1979) also suggested that the typical distinction between psychotherapy and counseling becomes quite blurred when working with older people. Therefore, although theoretically counseling and psychotherapy often have different goals, in actual practice with the elderly, counseling resembles psychotherapy more closely than the multitude of behavioral, environmental techniques adopted mostly for use with institutionalized elderly persons.

The techniques variously described as *reality, milieu,* or *resocialization therapy* all have much in common (Gilbert, 1977). They generally attempt to enlist the aid of various disciplines to restructure the functioning of ward personnel and manipulate environmental procedures to improve behavioral functioning and increase awareness of the external world. Gilbert (1977) cited studies which employed a variety of such techniques in diverse settings and reported improvement in both patients' adaptive functioning and staff morale (Bok, 1971; Burnside, 1971; Gottesman, et al., 1973). The utility of such procedures has been questioned, however, in studies which found that measured improvement occured only under specific conditions and did not generalize to other aspects of functioning (Bok, 1971; Brody, Kleban, Lawton & Silverman, 1971).

With psychotherapy defined, the question of whether such procedures can alleviate emotional problems and improve functioning of the elderly can be discussed. Unfortunately, there is not a large body of research which systematically evaluates psychotherapy outcome with the elderly. In the main, this has been due to a lack of interest on the part of many therapists in working with the elderly (Butler, 1975). Another factor has been the characteristic reluctance of the aged individual to seek mental health services due to ignorance, suspicion and shame (Kastenbaum, 1978).

Butler & Lewis (1973) noted that although individual psychotherapy is least available to the elderly, they often exhibit a strong drive to resolve problems and demonstrate a capacity for change. These authors suggested that there is very little empirical evidence that the elderly are untreatable. Based on their clinical experience, they found that elderly persons without brain damage are receptive to psychotherapy and should not be ruled out as candidates for treatment. These authors also advocated that all forms of psychotherapy may be used to come to a better understanding of the existential crises and adaptive processes involved in the psychology of old age. Ingebretson (1977), in her comprehensive discussion of psychotherapy with the elderly, also addressed the question of whether the elderly are amenable to such interventions. She concluded that age per se does not preclude a client's willingness or motivation to change; she, in fact, suggested that parallels exist between the existential crises of both young and elderly persons. Not only do the elderly face problems which are amenable by psychotherapy, but such therapy affords an opportunity to study and resolve issues related to the conclusion of the life cycle.

A major related issue concerns the capacity of the elderly to change. Pessimism about the ability of the elderly to make significant personality change has persisted since the beginnings of psychoanalysis, and has served to block initiation of therapeutic contracts with the elderly (Brink, 1977, 1979; Ingebretson, 1977; Rechtschaffen, 1959; Wilensky & Weiner, 1977). Freud stated that beyond age fifty individuals lack the flexibility and mental capacity necessary to learn or achieve insight in therapy. As Cath (1972) pointed out, subsequent analysts disagreed with Freud over this issue. Abraham (1949) conducted successful psychoanalysis with several older individuals, and warned against using any particular age as a criterion for successful therapy. He argued that the age of the neurosis is a more important predictor of outcome than the age of the patient. Indeed, a large body of research suggests there is no predictive relationship between age of patient and therapy outcome (Cabeen & Coleman, 1962; Cartwright, 1955; Feifel & Ellis, 1963; Liederman, Green & Liederman, 1967; Rosenbaum, Friedlander & Kaplan, 1956; Seeman, 1954). Wilensky & Weiner (1977) have suggested that many of the difficulties and poor results attributed to psychotherapy with the aged actually result from attempting psychotherapy with nonpsychologically minded adults who are poor candidates for traditional psychotherapeutic methods regardless of age. In a similar vein, Blum & Tallmer (1977) decry the lack of studies on procedure and techniques and point out that pessimistic evaluations of psychotherapy with the elderly are inevitable because much of the gerontological research has been conducted in nursing homes and veterans hospitals with a chronic, institutionalized, "captive" population which is atypical of most elderly individuals.

Although Fenichel (1945) shared Freud's pessimistic outlook for treatment of the elderly through classic analysis, he nonetheless felt that therapy is not altogether impossible beyond age forty, particularly if modifications were introduced. More recently, other theorists in the dynamic analytic tradition (Gitelson, 1965; Goldfarb, 1955; Grotjahn, 1955; Kaufman, 1940;

Meerloo, 1955; Rosenthal, 1959; Wayne, 1952; Wolff, 1963) have reported success in therapy and described deep-seated changes among elderly clients using modified psychoanalytic techniques. Rosenthal (1959) stated that conceptions of the elderly as lacking the desire or capability to change and as being satisfied with the status quo come from prejudicial cultural stereotypes. He concluded from his work with thirty patients ages fifty-eight to seventy-two that, although certain neurotic preoccupations and defenses can become more pronounced with the passage of time, these individuals could become as deeply involved in therapy as younger clients. Brink (1977) noted that over two-thirds of Jung's (1973) patients were considered elderly, and that Jung considered psychotherapy an effective tool for promoting psychic growth. The emphasis placed by Jungian therapy on the role of introspection, symbols and religion makes it a highly useful vehicle for the exploration of dynamics inherent in the aging process.

Related to the effectiveness of psychotherapy with the elderly is the question of whether the elderly generally can be motivated to change. Ingerbretson (1977) indicated that such motivation can rise from the experience of distress and hope for change that often accompanies advancing age. The elderly are frequently considered unmotivated, resistant to change, and therefore unresponsive to psychotherapy. Statistics show that relatively few older persons actively seek therapy. The highest frequency of suicide in males apparently occurs between the ages of sixty and seventy (Knight, 1979; Sparacino, 1979). Other writers (Butler, 1975; Kastenbaum, 1978) think that such reasoning is illogical and unwarranted, and they explain the lack of active participation and open investment in therapy as a reaction against the stigma attached to being old (senility, uselessness, etc.). This is coupled with their natural tendency to withdraw and become more internalized. Another reason may be that the elderly are affected by the general prejudice against admitting to emotional disorders.

Brink (1979) contradicted this presumed lack of motiviation by indicating that the elderly possess maturity and common sense, and are motivated by a great sense of urgency to achieve the maximal amount of satisfaction and adjustment in the time remaining to them. Other writers (Berezin, 1972; Butler & Lewis, 1973; Rosenthal, 1959) also emphasized that the motivation of the elderly for change can actually be stronger than that observed in the young, because of their acute awareness of the passage of time. The older person may feel a strong responsibility to work for change and a need to come to terms with the past and present in order to achieve understanding and acceptance of life.

Support for this idea takes the form of several outcome studies of psychotherapy successes which indicate that, although the elderly are least likely to seek treatment, they are far more likely to benefit from therapy than are college students (Sparacino, 1970). Estimates of the effectiveness of psychotherapy among older patients range from 50 to 80 percent treatment successes (Stonecypher, 1974). Although there are relatively few systematic, methodologically rigorous outcome studies to provide solid evidence for the effectiveness of psychotherapy with the elderly, numerous reports from practicing clinicians attest to the value of using psychotherapy to achieve beneficial results in elderly clients. For example, Blau & Berezin (1975), Busse (1971), and Cumming & Cumming (1975) have reported successful treatment of emotionally disturbed, elderly clients manifesting a variety of psychopatho-

logical symptoms using psychotherapy. Numerous
clinicians (Brink, 1979; Goldfarb, 1971; Karpf, 1980)
agreed that use of brief psychotherapy is quite effective
with older persons. Hiatt (1971, 1975), Langley (1975),
and Pfeiffer (1971) noted the effectiveness of dynamic
psychotherapy in the expression and alleviation of
symptoms. Radebold (1976) and Verwoerdt (1976)
reported success using psychoanalytic group psychotherapy with the elderly. Others (Howells, 1975; Peterson, 1973) have extended principles of family therapy
and achieved success in treatment of the elderly.

In short, it can hardly be concluded that psychotherapy is impossible or impractical with older people.
Numerous writers in the field (Butler, 1975; Davis &
Klopfer, 1977; Gilbert, 1977; Ingebretson, 1977; Karpf,
1977; Kastenbaum, 1978) have argued that ultimately,
doubts about the utility of psychotherapy with the
elderly reflect the value systems of society and the
personal orientations of therapists. The elderly in our
society comprise a very heterogeneous group. They
exhibit both diversity and individuality in coping abilities, life-styles, personality, physical health and expression of emotional problems. It is impractical therefore to generalize about *age* and the utility of psychotherapy. It is important however to maintain therapeutic flexibility and open-mindedness in working with
the elderly and to lay to rest devaluations of psychotherapy with older people which only serve to impede
progress in adapting successful interventions for them.

Ultimately, questions concerning the utility of traditional psychotherapy with the elderly must be asked in
light of the widespread and efficacious use of antidepressant medication in alleviating much of the suffering caused by depression. Since the effects of the tricyclic antidepressants were first described in the 1950's, a

number of controlled double-blind studies have substantiated their value in treatment of depressions, particularly those which are considered severe, psychotic and/or endogenous, but with more reactive neurotic depressions as well (Fann, 1976). Weissman (1978) has made the valid observation that psychotherapy should never be carried out to the exclusion of pharmacological intervention if the latter is warranted. Although Kral (1976) has supported the view that pharmacological therapy is the preferred treatment for endogenous, psychotic depression in the elderly, he also argued that psychotherapy should be considered the treatment of choice in the neurotic, situational depressions of late life. Blank (1974) likewise agreed that, because depression is an almost routine concomitant of the aging process, psychotherapy should be the treatment of choice, with medication used primarily to deal with crisis precipitated by severe and protracted depression such as suicidal behavior.

Another medication recently found useful in the treatment of recurrent, unipolar depressive illness and acute psychotic depression is lithium (Davis, 1976). Cox, Pearson & Brand (1977) suggested that use of lithium with the elderly be predicated on diagnosis of bipolar affective illness or frequently recurring, unipolar depressions. It is interesting to note that even the treatment of such supposedly endogenous, psychotic, genetically determined affective disorders may be improved by the simultaneous use of psychotherapy. Benson (1975) has provided outcome data on 31 cases with bipolar illness which shows psychotherapy in conjunction with lithium therapy achieved better results than did lithium therapy alone.

Lipton (1976) cautioned that, regardless of age, the causes of depression are multiple and not fully understood at present. Although the current concepts of the biological pathogenesis of depression all contain serious flaws, Lipton (1976) noted that evidence based upon the mechanism of action of antidepressant drugs does offer indirect evidence that depression is associated with alterations in the synthesis, storage, release, utilization and degradation of chemical neurotransmitters. Furthermore, alterations in the actions of enzymatic systems mediating these mechanisms are genetically programmed and occur as a function of the aging process. Thus, Lipton (1976) explained the increased prevalence and incidence of depression in the elderly in terms of the interaction between biological and psychosocial changes, and suggested that although the effects of anti-depressant treatment are usually notable, these may often require further potentiation in conjuction with appropriate, supportive psychosocial interventions (i.e., psychotherapy).

Gerner (1979) noted that pharmacotherapy and other somatic therapies such as electroconvulsive therapy have a primary role in treatment of affective disorders. He cited research showing that although 20 percent of depressions do not readily respond, true treatment-resistant cases are uncommon and may reflect lack of a thorough trial of various antidepressant medications. Nevertheless, Karpf (1980) preferred to describe pharmacotherapy as a "biochemical adjunct" to psychotherapy. Karpf (1980) argued that pharmacotherapy does not offer a true cure or heal emotional problems the way antibiotics cure an infection, but rather that such interventions maintain the impression of a cure by masking the symptoms of the disorder. Karpf (1980) also deplored the logic suggesting that, because illnesses such as depression or schizophrenia are thought to have a biochemical etiology, only biochemical treatments can permanently alter the disease process. He suggested that it is quite possible for environmental, exogenous treatments (i.e., psychotherapy) to produce the physiological changes related to improvement in depression discussed by Lipton (1976).

Several outcome studies have been conducted to further assess the relative effectiveness of pharmacological and psychotherapeutic interventions in depression (Covi, Lipman, Derogatis, Smith & Pattison, 1974; Friedman, 1975; Klerman, DiMascio, Weissman, Prusoff & Paykel, 1974; Lipman & Covi, 1976; Lipman, Covi & Smith, 1975; Weissman, Klerman, Paykel, Prusoff & Hanson, 1974). These studies have consistently shown that antidepressant medications significantly relieve depression, that subjects relapse if medication is discontinued, and that psychotherapy has little or no effect on symptoms or relapse. Conversely, these studies have also generally concluded that psychotherapy does have a positive effect on aspects of social function, attitudes and interpersonal relationships, while only one reported similar effects due to medication (Weissman, 1978).

However, these findings have recently been questioned because of several controlled, comparison outcome studies (Kovacs, Rush, Beck & Hollon, 1981; Rounsaville, Klerman & Weissman, 1981; Rush, Beck, Kovacs, & Hollon, 1977; Weissman, Prusoff, DiMascio, Neu, Goklaney & Klerman, 1979) which have suggested that the combination of psychological and pharmacological treatment is more effective than either used separately. Kovacs (1980) has, in fact, noted that, in some cases, psychotherapy in the form of social-skills training and cognitive interventions may even exceed drug treatment in both symptom-reduction and treatment-completion rate.

It appears that the use of medications constitutes an effective and prudent treatment in most cases of moderate to severe depression, regardless of precipitating factors or etiological classification. Despite this apparent success, there are many important considerations with regard to use of drugs with the elderly—considerations that render the traditional psychotherapy approach more attractive. Gerner (1979) observed that special precautions must be followed when instituting drug therapy of any kind for the elderly. The elderly do not have the same responses to medicines as do young persons (Fann, 1976; Friedel, 1980). There are alterations in absorption, storage, binding and excretion rates and mechanisms (Verwoerdt, 1976).

Salzman & Shader (1978a) examined the possible role that the simultaneous over-prescription of various medications (i.e., polypharmacy) may play in exacerbating depressions in the elderly. It is their contention that, regardless of whether or not they are prescribed by a physician for the treatment of medical or psychiatric disorders, drugs may often lead to the development of depression, exacerbation of pre-existing depressions, or production of depression-like symptoms in the elderly. Some medications commonly prescribed for the elderly (digitalis, antihypertensive agents, particularly reserpine and methyldopa, L-Dopa, corticosteroids and various neuroleptic preparations) can also interact to produce depressive symptoms (Salzman & Shader, 1978a). These authors also presented evidence suggesting that, in rare instances, it is possible that anti-depressant medications may themselves increase depressive symptoms. Finally, Gerner (1979) and others (Brink, 1977; Fann, 1976; Kral, 1976; Verwoerdt, 1976) felt compelled to point out the numerous, potentially dangerous, side effects associated with tricyclic antidepressant medications. These may include precipitation of glaucoma, urinary obstruction, hypotension and cardiac arrhythmias, as well as inducement of acute psychotic states including mania. These authors generally agreed that proper introduction and judicious maintenance of the drug regimens are necessary. There must be skillful monitoring by competent physicians who are thoroughly grounded in the specialized field of geriatric medicine.

It is important to emphasize that the disadvantages and dangers in the pharmacotherapy of depression do not negate the evidence of its effectiveness. These aspects were discussed only to point out that no form of therapy is a panacea, and that one cannot risk the development of a "magic bullet" mentality. As discussed in preceding sections, attitudinal biases and negativism towards the elderly have been rampant. Drug taking, especially when it involves emotional disorders, becomes stigmatizing. It is true for the general population and often for the medical (non psychiatric) community; therefore; the true danger lies in general population and often for the medical (nonpsychiatric) community; therefore, the true danger lies in the potential exacerbation of these attitudes through cated, the key to successful psychotherapy with the elderly lies in comprehensive medical, psychological and sociological assessment and interventions involving the combined efforts of a multi-disciplinary treatment network.

CHAPTER III

DIFFERENTIAL DIAGNOSIS

Epstein (1976) noted that although depression is quite common in the elderly, it is often overlooked or misdiagnosed. Its heterogeneous nature often results in diagnostic confusion and improper treatment.

To promote awareness of their implications for the conduct of psychotherapy with elderly persons, some problems of differential diagnosis and certain philosophical questions should be discussed. Differential diagnosis, as used here, differs from mere diagnosis in that it attempts to sort out finer variations within a syndrome.

Overlap of Depression with Other Emotional and Physical Problems

According to Lippincott (1968) and Goldstein (1979) the diagnosis of depression in the elderly typically involves criteria applied to all age groups. This includes depressive affect or mood, insomnia, anorexia and weight loss, apathy, fatigue, guilt and somatic preoccupations. They cautioned however that these symptoms may be highly varied and are often masked by the aging process and associated with environmental changes. Several authors (Epstein, 1976; Goldstein, 1979; Jarvik, 1976) have strongly emphasized that a satisfactory diagnostic classification scheme of depression has yet to be developed. Jarvik (1976) noted that the lack of an adequate nosology raises important philosophical and practical questions regarding etiology and treatment of depression, such as whether an initial onset of depression in late life is in any way different from depression that occurs for the first time earlier in life. Although current diagnostic criteria are less than adequate, it is extremely important not only to recognize the symptoms of depression but to be aware of the overlap between depression and other physical and emotional disorders.

In their comprehensive review, Salzman & Shader (1979) pointed out that, although depression in the elderly may often share many characteristics of the disorder found in younger individuals, the aged are more likely to resort to a variety of ego-defense mechanisms to distort or mask depressive symptoms. These may include use of denial, counterphobic defenses or somatization. These processes can make the recognition and evaluation of depression more difficult in the elderly because adaptive ego-defenses that were often employed successfully earlier in life may, in later years, become exaggerated or less resilient, and their original function or purpose may be transformed by changed life-circumstances. The defensive coping mechanism of denial is perhaps most common in the elderly and may account, in large part, for the failure to recognize both physical and emotional problems (Busse & Pfeiffer, 1973; Butler & Lewis, 1973). Somatization is a defense in which psychological problems such· as depression are expressed as bodily symptoms. Through this process, depressive affect may be disguised so that the individual does not consciously experience it. Verwoerdt (1976) has argued that somatic preoccupations have the advantage of helping the older individual avoid feelings of despair and the responsibility of dealing with real or imagined inadequacies.

Somatization and hypochondriacal complaints are extremely common in the elderly and often provide the therapist with the only clues to the existence of underlying depression (Busse, 1976; Busse & Pfeiffer, 1973). When such complaints occur during a time of life normally associated with physical decline and disease, the underlying depression may become extremely difficult to detect. Repeated physical complaints (often involving the gastrointestinal system) may be a sign of depression. Vegetative signs of depression (apathy, decreased energy, etc.) are important diagnostically because they often provide early warning that depressive illness is underway.

Salzman & Shader (1979) suggested that differential diagnosis of depressions having a medical or physiological origin and those having a psychogenic origin is often difficult. This is because apathy, insomnia, decreased energy, pain, somatic symptoms and hypochondriasis all may signify depression as well as medical disease. Physical illness frequently precipitates or accompanies depression (Pfeiffer & Busse, 1973). Busse (1965) suggested the deterioration in physical functioning is more likely to precipitate a reactive depression in the elderly than loss of loved ones or loss of self-esteem. Verwoerdt (1976) stated that the extent of depressive response to physical illness in the elderly depends upon the severity, duration and rate of progression of the physical illness. He argued that depression varied with the amount of the individual's narcissistic attachment to the physical capabilities altered by the disease process. Salzman & Shader (1979) noted that severe depressive reactions to physical illness in the elderly are common, particularly in the case of cardiovascular disease and cancer. These authors observed that although patients with chronic disease may suffer from reactive depressions regardless of age, the elderly constitute a particularly vulnerable group.

Salzman & Shader (1979) observed that not only can physical disease coincide with or precipitate depression or depressive-like symptoms, but that depression itself may be expressed by a variety of physical symptoms. The indirect expression of depression through primarily physical mechanisms has been termed *depressive equivalent* or *masked depression* (Butler & Lewis, 1973; Pfeiffer & Busse, 1973). Nowlin & Busse (1977) noted that psychosomatic disorders in the elderly are often maintained by a concurrent depression, and therefore, treatment of chronic musculoskeletal back and neck pain with antidepressant drugs often results in gradual diminution of symptoms along with lifting of depression. Conversely, many elderly patients who are suffering from acute depression are often initially treated for a pre-existing physical disorder.

The relationship between hypochondriasis and

depression is widely accepted (Epstein, 1976; Fann, 1976; Jarvik, 1976; Pfeiffer & Busse, 1973). In such cases the individual may appear depressed yet consistently deny it. According to Epstein (1976) most elderly persons who display this pattern suffer from neurotic or reactive-type depressions, often in response to environmental deprivations and/or physical decline. They often reveal a history of previous neurotic personality traits, particularly obsessive or compulsive patterns (Wolff, 1977). Thus hypochondriasis can immeasureably complicate the differential diagnosis of depression in the elderly.

The overlap between depression and various chronic, degenerative, organic brain syndromes constitutes another source of difficulty frequently found in the differential diagnosis of depression in the elderly. Eisdorfer & Cohen (1978) point out that, while in theory chronic brain diseases and depression present distinguishable clinical pictures, in practice they are often difficult to separate, because depression often accompanies the cognitive and physical changes associated with chronic brain syndromes. Whitehead (1974) stated that many symptoms and behaviors presumed to be signs of irreversible, organically based deterioration in the elderly may actually represent underlying, unrecognized depressions which often respond dramatically to treatment. Raskind & Eisdorfer (1976) noted that approximately nine percent of those referred to a treatment program on the basis of cognitive disorders (i.e., senile dementia) actually exhibited a clinical depression.

Epstein (1976) observed that depression is often easily mistaken for a progressive, chronic brain dysfunction, because when depression is severe or left untreated long enough, the resulting marked psychomotor retardation, memory deficiency and cognitive impairment may closely simulate senile dementia. This form of depression is often referred to as "pseudodementia" (Busse & Pfeiffer, 1973; Verwoerdt, 1976) but may be reliably distinguished from true dementia by a relatively short history of symptoms, previous personal or family history of depression, and inconsistencies in the expression of the cognitive and intellectual impairment (Epstein, 1976). Fann & Wheless (1975) also report that worsening depression is so often associated with the slowing of intellective processes and psychomotor retardation that moderate to severe depression with minimal organic involvement is often misdiagnosed as chronic brain disease such as cerebral arteriosclerosis or senile dementia. These authors suggested several means of differentiating functional depressions from depressions secondary to brain disease. While functional or psychogenic depressions are usually marked by a more abrupt onset, organically based depressions are less precipitous, with milder, insidious early symptoms that fluctuate and finally disappear as the organic deterioration progresses (Fann & Wheless, 1975).

As Karpf (1977) observed, differentiation between the primary organic disorder and the salient but secondary depressive condition is often very complex and has important implications for treatment. Karpf (1977) maintained that when depression is secondary to a medical disease, it should be treated medically. In those cases where the depression is thought to involve *both* the disease process and unsuccessful compensatory coping mechanisms, Karpf (1977) argued that environmental interventions, such as psychotherapy, are indicated. He thought that this reasoning may draw an overly fine line. The inherent danger is the presumption that once a diagnosis of organic depression is made, psychotherapy in such cases will be unproductive. Karpf (1977) warned against adopting this line of reasoning. Goldfarb (1974) vehemently attacked this logic and provided considerable evidence of the utility of therapy with older persons with this type of problem. The next section illustrates that, because practically all affective changes, whether organically or environmentally based, inevitably reflect an interaction between aging, internal and external stressors and individual personality dynamics, psychotherapy must always be considered a viable treatment option.

Interaction between Aging, Life Stress, Personality and Mood Change

Epstein (1976) argued for the need to acknowledge the role played by many interacting facts in the culmination of late-life depressions. These include the individual's lifelong experiences, current environment, changing physical status and other stresses impinging upon emotional adjustment. Epstein (1976) observed that emotional well-being in the elderly was primarily affected by age-related stresses, hereditary factors, and premorbid personality. Thus, he concluded that a single and primary source of depressive illness was improbable. Defining the phenomenon as interactional, Epstein (1976) supported the contention that depression represents the final, common pathway for a multitude of biological, social and environmental variables (Akiskal, 1978; Akiskal & McKinney, 1975). The implication inherent in this approach is that depression may respond to a variety of different intervention strategies and that any therapy of depression in the elderly must be responsive to these factors.

Klerman (1976) expressed dissatisfaction with the ambiguities of diagnostic labels and the lack of sufficient data to permit adequate classification of depression in terms of distinctive personality patterns. He argued, for example, that the concept of reactive depression based upon reaction to stressful life events is a serious oversimplification. To be considered truly comprehensive, an account of depression must describe the interaction between individual predisposing constitutional factors, early personality development, and adjustments necessitated by environmental demands for adaptive change (Klerman, 1972, 1976). Jarvik (1976) supported this and suggested that the appearance of depression in late life depends upon the severity and number of stresses relative to the adaptive capacity of the individual. Stresses may have a physical, chemical, intrapsychic or psychosocial origin, while adaptive capacity may have both biological and psychological determinants.

With regard to particular personality dispositions possibly predictive of depression, individuals who tend to perceive and evaluate their environment negatively are considered more likely to develop depression (Beck, 1976; Lunghi, 1977). Stresses of all kinds may be integrated or may cause disintegration depending upon their quantity and quality in conjunction with the individual's unique personality, for it is personality that determines vulnerability to specific threat or loss. Gerner (1979) presented evidence that certain personality characteristics are associated with depression. Rigid personalities and compulsives tend to have a greater chance of developing depressive affect and behaviors (Kendell & Discipio, 1970; Wolff, 1970). This personality type is typically held to have psychogenic roots, but it may also be inherited (Woodruff, Goodwin & Guze, 1974). It is also plausible that individuals with narcissistic qualities and those where self-concept depends on qualities that deteriorate with age are particularly vulnerable to depression in late life (Gerner, 1979).

Jarvik (1976) has acknowledged that many questions pertaining to the qualitative similarity of depression across the age continuum remain unanswered. She also observed that answers to these questions would probably vary with the type and nature of depressive disorder and the adaptative capacity of the individual. Gurland (1976) also noted that adaptation in later years often involves causal factors related to depression, including significant life events, work and retirement patterns, family and social relationships, chronic physical disease, and that all of these can synergistically influence biological, age-related changes in metabolic processes.

Busse & Pfeiffer (1973) also related current adaptive functioning to an interweaving of biological, social and psychological factors impinging upon the individual. They further contended that adaptive functioning in the elderly reflects both uniqueness and continuity with other stages of the life cycle. Thus old age represents a unique phase with different problems, tasks and limitations than found in earlier years. Nevertheless, the fundamental style the individual uses to handle these concerns ensures a remarkable degree of continuity with patterns established in early life.

Qualitative Similarity of Depression
across the Life Span

The final diagnostic and etiological issue to be discussed in this section is whether depression in later life may be viewed as qualitatively and/or phenomenoloically similar to early onset depressions. This question has profound implications for the way depression in the elderly is viewed. It directly influences the way psychotherapy is conducted with this population. Several important related questions also evolve from a consideration of this issue, such as whether depression ever should be regarded as an inevitable consequence of the aging process. Another issue is whether depression ever should be judged as representing a realistic appraisal of, and adjustment to, the diminished status, roles and capacities accompanying advancing age.

The question of the qualitative similarity of depression across the life span reflects two divergent theoretical traditions. By its overemphasis on the importance of early life as *the* determinant of personality, early psychoanalytic theory led to a disregard of the importance of the problems and stresses that are unique to later stages of the life span (Cath, 1978). Neugarten (1973) noted that traditional analytic theory has provided few concepts with which to comprehend post-adolescent personality change. The analytic view is basically that, once one's personal sense of identity is forged, consistency in behavior follows along with fixation of character structure. One important exception among early analytic theorists in this regard was Jung (Brink, 1979; Neugarten, 1973; Verwoerdt, 1976). Jung (1973) described stages of adult development and worked with individuals over age fifty. He observed a trend toward increased introversion with passage of time and characterized adulthood and later life as a time of reorganization of value systems.

Erikson was another analytically based theorist who broke with traditional views. He extended the domain of personality development across the life span, and delineated eight stages, each of which involves a choice point of life crisis for the individual. In the last stage (integrity versus despair) the individual is faced with the task of reviewing and assessing past accomplishments. Successful resolution and adaptation to old age thus requires a satisfactory evaluation of preceding life history. As Brink (1979) observed however, this model is often of little value to the psychotherapist because it does not confront the current, urgent biological, psychological and social crises of later life. Brink (1979) argued that the most salient psychopathology in the elderly is not existential despair brought about by a review of past failures but reactive-type depressions triggered by current life events and changes. Busse & Pfeiffer (1973) stated that Erikson's theory emphasized both the uniqueness of each phase of the life cycle as well as its essential continuity with all other phases. Although Erikson (1959, 1968) intended to dramatize continuity through the ongoing successful resolution of age-appropriate conflicts presented by successive life stages, his model may have inadvertently fostered the illusion that personality organization and expression of psychopathology is qualitatively different across the different stages. This confusion may be due to the structure of the model itself, which outlines different themes at different stages of life.

Others have also argued that it may be more parsimonious to view the emotional problems of older persons as qualitatively similar to those of younger individuals, and that instead of overemphasizing differences based upon chronological age, one should focus upon the specific problems of the client (Brink, 1979; Kastenbaum, 1978; Neugarten, 1973; Vickers, 1976). One implication of this for psychotherapy is that specific techniques that have been developed for particular disorders may be used with the expectation that they will achieve similar results regardless of the age of the client. Kastenbaum (1978), in particular, strongly endorsed this approach. He suggested that the elderly person who is struggling with massive transitions in life may be more similar to young adults also facing dramatic role adjustment and life change than to same-age persons who are less uprooted. Kastenbaum (1978) noted that depression is a problem that is by no means limited to the aged, and that using existing theory and therapy dealing with depression may be more effective than trying to develop a special theory exclusively for use with the elderly. Kastenbaum (1978) indicated that both the nature of the particular emotional problem and the specific characteristics and dynamics of the individual should determine the focus of therapy, and not the person's chronological age.

Neugarten (1973) contended that old age represents neither separate nor discontinuous periods in the life cycle. Old age may have unique characteristics, but it is enmeshed in the same system of biological and sociocultural influences that determine behavior and adaptation at all ages. Because personality factors reflect long-standing life-styles, this view maintains that patterns of coping continue as the individual passes into old age. Although there may be no single, prescribed pattern or scenario by which people age, they seem to exhibit continuity by adapting over time, in ways that are consistent with patterns established in younger years. The coping behavior of older persons is therefore similar to younger persons and reflects choices that are most consonant with long established, stable values and self-concepts (Brink, 1979; Neugarten, 1973). This model suggests that those individuals who typically reacted to stresses in early life by becoming depressed are more likely to manifest similar behaviors when confronted with the increasing adaptational requirements and stresses imposed by the aging process. Busse & Pfeiffer (1973) agreed that adaptation in early life is probably the best predictor of adaptation in old age. In support of this, they cited evidence that those who developed emotional problems in late life tended to exhibit more maladjustments in early life, whereas people who exhibit successsful adaptation in old age generally have been well-adjusted throughout their lives.

Evidence supporting the qualitative similarity of depression across the age continuum comes from numerous sources. Pfeiffer & Busse (1973) observed that older persons may manifest any of the psychiatric disorders found in younger adults, and argued that treatment for severe depression in old age is not qualitatively different from the treatment of these disorders in younger persons. Gilbert (1977) agreed with this premise and felt that most older persons respond to psychotherapy as well as younger persons, regardless of type of therapy used. Raskin (1979) maintained that, even if one accepts the premise that the elderly are particularly susceptible to physical and psychosocial factors that can precipitate depression, it does not necessarily signify that depression manifests itself differently in older people than in younger ones. In his review, Raskin (1979) called for further research efforts to clarify and document differences in the frequency, quality and intensity of depression in both younger and older adults.

Vickers (1976) stated that mental impairment is not an inevitable product of old age. He cited Donahue (1971) who stressed that both the physical and emotional disabilities of the elderly are not different in kind from those encountered in younger persons; the difference lies with the patient and not the pathology. Feigenbaum (1974) also stressed the qualitative similarity of depression in all age groups, and stated that the elderly were no less prone to particular crises in adaptation than younger individuals. Ingebretson (1977) maintained that depression in the elderly may be quite similar to earlier onset depressions because they frequently represent a direct continuation of the same neurotic defenses and coping styles previously erected by the individual. This supports the view that personality traits persist across the life span. Krasner (1977) noted that aging is a continuum in which underlying character structure remains relatively intact in spite of increasing variability in manner of adaptive functioning and expression of symptomatology. Taking this qualitative similarity and constancy into account, Davis and Klopfer (1977) indicated that it is quite feasible to use the same methods of psychotherapy in treating depressions and adjustment problems regardless of the age of the individual.

To summarize, there has been considerable debate over the issue of whether depression is qualitatively and existentially similar or dissimilar across the life span. The authors of this book contend that these two views are not irreconcilable. The experience of depression is probably qualitatively similar at every age. Furthermore, the form of the external and internal stress factors precipitating depression may also be similar. What seems different is that old age may be associated with an ever-increasing *accumulation* of stresses which may overwhelm the adaptive capacity of the individual. Although age adds a quantitative element, subjective experience and expression of depressive symptoms remain relatively constant. When viewed this way, the two apparently divergent views discussed above (Erikson, 1959, 1968 and Neugarten, 1973) are reconcilable.

As alluded to above, advancing age is accompanied by unique adaptational challenges that may contribute to the development of depression. These may take the form of various psychosocial, biological and environmental stresses, all of which are characterized primarily by some kind of loss. The next section focuses on the role these losses play in depression, and briefly examines the phenomenon of disengagement as a concomitant of the aging process. Disengagement may constitute a defensive maneuver or coping strategy in older persons faced with progressive cumulative life stress, losses and physical decline.

CHAPTER IV

FACTORS ASSOCIATED
WITH LATE-LIFE DEPRESSIONS

SOCIAL FACTORS AND
ENVIRONMENTAL PROCESSES

Loss

Numerous authors have suggested that loss is an inherent part of the aging process and a frequent theme in the emotional experience of the elderly (Butler & Lewis, 1973; Charatan, 1975; Palmore, 1973). Both dynamic and behavioral formulations of depression attach significant importance to the role played by

37

losses in the etiology of depression (Busse & Pfeiffer, 1977; Fann & Wheless, 1975; Lewinsohn, 1975; Verwoerdt, 1976). Loss figures heavily in Butler & Lewis' (1973) description of the complex interaction of extrinsic and intrinsic factors affecting level of adaptation in the elderly. These include personal losses such as the death of one's spouse, close friends and other family members, and social losses, such as loss of prestige due to retirement, or the loss of self-esteem due to cultural devaluation of the aging. Finally, the ongoing loss of physical powers associated with the aging process can also contribute to despair as the individual becomes increasingly aware of the inevitability of death.

According to Peck (1966), the elderly are particularly vulnerable to stresses induced by losses in both the biological and socioeconomic spheres. It has been well documented that physical declines such as loss of muscular strength, coordination, reflex speed and sensory acuity are accepted as a normal consequence of aging (Birren, 1964; Botwinick, 1973). In addition to these often subtle losses, the individual's physical appearance begins to deteriorate due to hormonal changes. Cognitive decline and intellectual changes are also noticed though they vary considerably from one person to the next. They may be the result of progressive arteriosclerosis or degenerative central nervous system processes. Peck (1966) also described the significant social and economic losses associated with aging in western culture, and suggested that the elderly person frequently suffers from the cumulative impact of loss of loved ones (parents, siblings, friends and children) who were significant sources of emotional support and continuity.

Peck (1966) and several subsequent authors (Goldfarb, 1974; Goldstein, 1979; Solomon, 1981) presented a model showing how losses could precipitate depression or other psychological illness. The basic assumption of this model is that biological, social and economic losses acting in concert result in a net decrease in mastery over the environment. While the perception of personal failures can be highly aversive to the elderly individual, the reduced frequency of positive experiences in interacting with the external world may further erode self-esteem. The natural reaction to these frustrations is fear and anger, both of which further disrupt ego-functioning, yielding additional decrements in adaptive capacity and creating a vicious circle of increasing helplessness, loss of self-esteem, despair and depression. Fann & Wheless (1975) supported this cyclical model of cumulative loss and stress as a major factor precipitating depression in the elderly. They cited research (Braceland, 1972; Carver, 1974) suggesting that the elderly are beset by increasingly adverse conditions at a time when their capacity to successfully cope and adapt is diminishing. The result is depression. Goldstein (1979) and Solomon (1981) further noted that negative societal stereotypes of the elderly, loss of mastery and control due to increased dependency, and culturally determined diminution of former roles, power, and status together produce a helplessness that leads to depression, anger, fear and anxiety.

In traditional Freudian theory, loss represents a deficiency of the external supplies needed to satisfy basic drives and needs (Levin, 1965; Verwoerdt, 1976). This view affirms that loss of someone loved or needed—someone in whom considerable narcissistic energy is invested or one who has been a source of gratification or emotional support—can be a precipitating factor in depression. Bibring (1953) noted the relationship between internal and external sources of loss and stress, the decline of physical capacities and adaptive skills, and defined depression as an emotional state characterized by the helplessness and powerlessness of the ego. According to Busse (1976), loss or fear of loss makes it increasingly difficult for the older person to reduce tension through need gratification. The resulting erosion of self-esteem and sense of competence can produce depressive mood states.

Salzman & Shader (1979) broadened the scope of loss to include decrease in any functional capacity, ability, skill or interpersonal relationship that had constituted a major source of love, pride, accomplishment, or in any way served the individual's needs. In this view, the concept of loss may embrace any manner of physical or cognitive decline, and it includes the loss of status and self-esteem associated with one's former role in society. Loss of employment or freedom of mobility may represent a serious threat to an older individual's sense of independence and pride, and lead to resignation, apathy, and further withdrawal and isolation. From a behavioral perspective, this withdrawal can easily be seen as a result of a significant decrease in the number and frequency of reinforcing events for the individual. In fact, the loss of significant reinforcers may be a major component in the etiology of depressive mood (Lewinsohn, 1975).

Gerner (1979), however, noted that, although aging is associated with an increased number of losses and stressors, this factor alone does not explain the occurrence of late onset depression in persons who previously were able to adapt to loss without becoming depressed. Furthermore, Gerner (1979) cited research showing that many older persons continue to adapt to multiple losses without exhibiting depression, and suggested that the effect of any particular stress or loss must always be evaluated within the context of individual personality variables.

In summary, it is evident that the aging process inevitably is accompanied by an escalation in both the number and different types of losses, many of which have no precedent in the individual's earlier life experiences. It seems warranted that these losses can have enough force to precipitate depression in the elderly, particularly in those persons whose self-concept is largely based upon qualities that naturally diminish with advancing age. It must be cautioned nevertheless, that due to variability of personality characteristics, there is no strict one-to-one correspondence between various losses and onset of depression (Bornstein, Clayton, Halikas, Maurice & Robins, 1973; Paykel, Myers, Dienelt, Klerman, Lindenthal & Pepper, 1969; Neiderehe, 1977). Furthermore, as Fassler & Gaviria (1978) observed, the elderly do not all experience and react to the viscissitudes of life in a similar way.

Disengagement

Disengagement has been discussed within the context of two opposing theoretical views. One view suggests that disengagement is a normal, adaptive coping response in the face of the multiple stressors impinging on the aging individual. The second view (activity theory) holds that disengagement is not good, normal or healthy and that the resulting social isolation often represents the beginning of emotional problems and personality disorganization. Disengagement theory was initially advanced as an outgrowth of the Kansas City longitudinal study of aging conducted by Cumming & Henry (1961). Based upon various indices of the life-satisfaction and social-activity level of a large sample, these authors maintained that decreased social interaction and participation demonstrated mutual withdrawal of the older person and society. Because the mutuality of this withdrawal was emphasized, it was proposed that in old age the individual who had disengaged successfully would have an enhanced sense of well-being and life satisfaction. As initially advanced by Cumming and Henry (1961), successful disengagement was held to be an inevitable developmental process involving either a reduction in the number of interactions expected of an individual in a given role, a reduction in the total number of roles required of the individual or a combination of both. According to Brink (1979) the positive correlation between disengagement and life satisfaction reflected the experience of freedom from burdens of prior social roles and commitments. The social withdrawal reflecting disengagement was felt to be preceded and/or accompanied by increased preoccupation with the self and decreased emotional investment in aspects of the external environment (Bell, 1978). As a consequence of this, psychological well-being in late life supposedly represented the attainment of a new equilibrium characterized by greater psychological distance, altered interpersonal relationships and decreased social interaction between the older person and the environment.

Disengagement theory has sparked intense debates in the field of social gerontology and geriatric psychology, and has been subject to intensive criticism, reformulation and modification. Indeed both Cumming (1963, 1964) and Henry (1965) attempted to enlarge the scope of the theory. Cumming (1964) discussed differential aspects of disengagement as they relate to social constraints, changing roles and biological differences such as temperament. Henry (1965) argued that disengagement was an intrinsic process, one that could not be accounted for solely on the basis of societal or environmental events, and that suitable explanations required analysis of personality dynamics as well. Nevertheless, criticism of the original disengagement theory emerged from a variety of sources (Glenwick & Whitbourne, 1977). The inevitability and positive adaptive function of disengagement has been questioned as has its ability to transcend different societal and cultural structures (Havinghurst, Neugarten & Tobin, 1968; Rose, 1964). The subsequent research showing adaptation at variance with that found by Cumming & Henry (1961) has called their sampling and procedural methods into question (Maddox, 1972). Furthermore, the basic trends of disengagement theory are also called into question by what is termed the activity theory of successful adaptation to aging.

As advanced by Havinghurst (1953, 1963), activity theory suggests that inevitable decrements in biological functioning notwithstanding, older persons are the same as the middle-aged, with virtually identical psychological and social needs. This view suggests that the increased social isolation in the elderly results from societal withdrawals from the aging person, and that this decreased social interaction runs counter to the desires of most aging individuals. Thus, activity theory holds that the hallmark of successful adaptation in late life is the individual who remains active, involved and who resists the erosion of middle-age capabilities as long as possible. In support of activity theory, Havinghurst, Neugarten, & Tobin, (1963), having analyzed the Kansas City data (Cumming & Henry, 1961), concluded that the more highly engaged individuals were with their environment and social roles the more likely they were to be well-adjusted and satisfied. An important implication for psychopatholgy is that depression would be less likely in those elderly persons who remain active and resist the withdrawal of society. It should be noted that both disengagement and activity theories agree that levels of activity and engagement decrease as people grow older. The key point of difference seems to reside in the claim by disengagement theorists that this reduction in social interaction is a mutual process and not merely the result of a unilateral withdrawal of society from the elderly person.

Neugarten (1968) further refined the disengagement theory and proposed a continuity theory which combined developmental and psychosocial processes in order to account for adjustment and successful aging. Neugarten (1973) proposed that individual differences are important in the ultimate pattern and sequence of disengagement in the elderly. Thus, the continuity view holds that successful aging and adaptation is ultimately dependent upon the continuation of enduring characteristics such as interests, cognitive style, drives, needs and behavioral patterns.

As Neugarten (1973) stated "disengagement proceeds at different rates and different patterns in different people in different places and has different outcomes with regard to psychological well-being." Neugarten concluded that disengagement theory is apparently accurate as a description of psychosocial processes, although it remains an inadequate account of all aspects of personality functioning or a universal description of successful aging. In recognition of these limitations, Glenwick & Whitbourne (1977) proposed a transactional model of disengagement that conceptualizes change and adaptation in late life as a dynamic interaction between past and present personality attributes influenced by both biological and psychosocial factors. Modifications in the level of adjustment of the aging person reflect an intricate pattern of interaction between unique personality and cognitive attributes, current environmental setting, and interpersonal transactions.

Despite continued research, the modifications and inconsistencies in the predictions generated from disengagement theory have clouded its status as a useful index of successful adaptation and life satisfaction among the elderly. Levin (1964) in particular has criticized some of the basic tenets of disengagement, most notably the idea that the withdrawal, self-centeredness, and isolation found among disengaged individuals is a routine by-product of the reduction of former social ties, responsibilities and burdens. Levin (1964) argued that the tranquility and contentment appearing in some disengaged persons may in fact disguise depression. In reality, the individual may experience apathy and narcissistic regression in response to loss, stress and threats to the integrity of the ego. Therefore it seems relevant to try to determine the extent to which underlying depression is actually the catalyst which promotes the disengagement process. Brink (1979) addressed this issue by suggestiong that the therapist needs to carefully analyze the type and extent of disengagement exhibited by the individual in order to discern the degree of the mutuality and intentionality of the isolation and withdrawal, i.e., the extent to which such isolation is a condition desired by the individual.

Disengagement may thus be viewed as the operation of selected ego-defense mechanisms in response to threat and changed life-circumstances. Numerous authors (Levin, 1964; Pfeiffer & Busse, 1973; Salzman

& Shader, 1979; Verwoerdt, 1976) have commented that adaptive ego-defenses enable the individual to retreat from threat, exclude it from awareness and enhance mastery and control over the environment. The withdrawal, isolation and reduced intensity of interactions with the environment that characterize the disengagement process may therefore serve a useful function. Nevertheless, adaptive ego-defenses employed in earlier years may become altered and exaggerated in response to changing life circumstances so that disengagement in the elderly could arguably be considered a maladaptive process leading to isolation, apathy and depression.

It seems quite likely that isolation may be a crucial factor in both disengagement and depression. Isolation can take on both interpersonal and intrapersonal qualities; thus it is possible to experience both social and psychological isolation, either of which may accompany or precipitate depression. Isolation is both intrinsic to and a by-product of the process of disengagement. Finally, isolation can represent an integral, adaptive, intrapsychic ego-defense. Nevertheless, self-imposed isolation to avoid negative feelings and the reluctance to share these feelings with family and friends may become counterproductive creating an insurmountable gulf that emotionally distances others and, ironically, weakens those affectional bonds most important in maintaining equilibrium (Zinberg & Kaufman, 1963). Indeed, Salzman & Shader (1979) have described disengagement as a progressive withdrawal from object relationships as affectional ties with significant others are severed. In this sense then, the elderly person who has disengaged may have become isolated both socially and affectively and is considerably more vulnerable to depression. This may explain how isolation could serve as one mechanism by which disengagement could lead to depression in older persons.

Based upon the limited research data available there is virtually no evidence to warrant the conclusion that depression is directly associated with or attributed to disengagement. However, evidence does exist that documents a certain relationship between social isolation (including interpersonal withdrawal and the attenuation of affectional relations) and intrapsychic defenses. Disengagement seems therefore to possess paradoxical qualities in that it is interpretable both as an adaptive ego-defense reaction that reduces stress to manageable levels in later life, enabling the individual to cope more effectively with change, *and* as a maladaptive pattern leading inexorably to isolation and depression. It is also important to note that disengagement was shown to be a function of both internal personality functioning and external, environmental or social factors.

PERSONALITY CONSTRUCTS
AND COGNITIVE PROCESSES

Rigidity

One of the more prominent personality characteristics typically ascribed to the elderly is that of rigidity. Rigidity, a result of presumed changes in the individual's manner of processing information or characteristic way of relating to the environment, has been invoked to explain behavior problems associated with aging.

It is said to be characterized by such behaviors and

attitudes as dogmatism, conservatism and unquestioning adherence to traditional values and beliefs (Botwinick, 1973; Brink, 1979). Operationally, this lack of flexibility has been defined as caution in high risk-reward situations, or reluctance to engage in creative new problem-solving approaches.

Although the elderly as a group have long been perceived as rigid, in part due to cultural stereotypes, both cross-sectional and longitudinal research clearly indicates that, even when potentially confounding variables such as IQ, socioeconomic status, education and health are controlled, the elderly as a group tend to exhibit greater rigidity on a variety of measures of this dimension. Botwinick (1973), however, cautioned that rigidity may be somewhat difficult to evaluate, because it may not be a unitary concept. Rigidity can assume many forms, not all of which are manifested by any one individual. This diffuse characteristic of rigidity, however, seems to call into question Botwinick's (1973) argument that rigidity is an inherent developmental process.

Brink (1979) preferred to view rigidity as a defensive mechanism used by the elderly in response to perceived threat or a hostile environment. Indeed, Neugarten (1969) found that the elderly tend to view the world as more complex and dangerous than younger individuals who typically exhibit a more exploitative and aggressive orientation towards the external environment. Rechtschaffen (1959) reported that rigidity may represent an adaptive ego-defense mechanism which could preserve and maintain a sense of equilibrium in the face of diminishing cognitive and sensory abilities. Early analytic theorists such as Jellifee (1925) and Kaufman (1940) argued that attempts to eliminate the rigid behavioral styles of some elderly individuals might actually undermine their level of functioning.

Considerable doubt remains about the precise relationship between rigidity and expressions of psychopathology among the aged. In particular, very little research has systematically explored the relationship between various manifestations of rigidity and late life depression. What little evidence exists does suggest that almost all measures of geriatric rigidity are correlated with poor adjustment (Havinghurst, 1957, 1963). Nevertheless, Brink (1978) argued that it is erroneous to assume that rigidity causes poor adjustment; rather, rigidity should be viewed as the elderly person's attempt to cope with increased physiological and social deficits. It appears that any disturbance, deviation or diminution of current level of functioning, whether gradual or precipitous, is capable of fostering rigid behavioral responses in particular individuals as a result of increased anxiety levels. This presupposes, of course, that the individual does in fact perceive the loss of functioning as a significant impairment. Thus, Brink (1979) suggested that anxiety and concerns about diminished functioning promote rigidity in the elderly. This often is evidenced by staunch adherence to old habits or problem-solving strategies and an unwillingness to experiment with altered behavior patterns despite feedback which suggests that the old strategies are ineffective.

With respect to the specific relationships, if any, between the rigidity of the older person and depressive mood, one plausible hypothesis is that rigidity directly stems from early-life deprivations, parental rejection or physical handicaps, and ultimately precipitates depression by blocking goal attainment and preventing individuals from actualizing their full potential

(Brink, 1979). By the same token, it could be argued that rigidity is merely a label given to describe any particularly inflexible adaptation made by an individual facing some major life stress or change, and it is these changes which are responsible for precipitating a depressive mood. Therefore, it is unclear whether rigidity causes depression in late life or is a by-product of forces which predispose the individual to depression. Perhaps the main reason for doubting that rigidity is a causal factor in depression is the observation that rigidity has been closely identified as a notable personality feature affecting the behaviors and cognitions of many elderly individuals, both depressed *and* nondepressed (Botwinick, 1973; Brink, 1979). Nevertheless, there is a smattering of research that suggests that individuals with rigid and/or obsessive-compulsive, premorbid personalities are more likely to express psychopathology in the form of depressive behavior and affect (Kendell & Discipio, 1970; Wolff, 1971). Although it would be premature to conclude that rigidity is a direct cause of depression, based upon current available research, it does seem plausible that the rigid personality is associated with the kinds of distorted cognitive processes and negative self-evaluations that have been implicated as determinants of depression (Beck, 1967, 1973; Lewinsohn, 1975; Seligman, 1975). In this context it becomes important to assess the degree of rigidity present in depressed elderly clients inasmuch as this determination will affect therapeutic intervention. Although rigidity, if present, may not directly cause depression and may not be found in all depressed individuals, it may represent the individual's attempt to cope with depression and consequently should be considered in discussions of what constitutes the most appropriate therapeutic strategy. Another personality variable with a somewhat more definitive and empirical relationship to depression is that of *locus of control*.

Locus of Control

Locus of control is the extent to which a person experiences outcomes as being contingent upon personal effort and abilities as opposed to being determined by chance or other external factors. It was first discussed by Rotter (1966) as one dimension of an individual's general expectancies. His view is that behavior is determined by needs and expectancies (both general and specific), and that these determinants come into play in different ways in different situations. Since its formulation by Rotter (1966), the concept of locus of control has received considerable attention because of its usefulness in accounting for relative levels of adjustment. Locus of control is an especially relevant and useful factor for assessing depression in the elderly, one that can provide a particularly valuable framework for use in therapy.

Reid, Haas & Hawkings (1977) contended that the locus of control concept affords insight into the analysis of psychological stresses associated with aging and with the adjustments the aging process demands from the individual. Research generally suggests that external locus of control beliefs are associated with a greater incidence of maladjustment as measured on self-report scales (Lefcourt, 1973; Strickland, 1973). Linn (1979) summarized most of this literature by noting that the salient differences between internal versus external locus of control individuals is that internals engage more frequently in instrumental, goal-directed activities, while externals are more likely to reveal negative affect-laden responses and non-goal directed activities. In addition to empirical findings, clinical experience supports the idea that loss of personal control over environmental contingencies and the lowered frequency of reinforcing events this produces often results in psychopathology characterized by a cyclical, maladaptive behavior pattern. Perhaps not surprisingly, Rotter (1966) argued that successful outcomes in therapy could be facilitated by attempting to orient individuals in the direction of internality.

The specific relationship between locus of control beliefs and adjustment in the elderly has received scant attention in the literature despite the contention of Reid et al. (1977) that changes in cognitive functioning may shift one's locus of control toward the external. This reduction in sense of personal effectiveness may then lead to expressions of psychopathology. Reid et al. (1977) acknowledged the tendency of changes in cognitive functioning to vary with changes in both the physical and social domain; nevertheless the precise parameters of this complex interaction have yet to be elucidated.

The available literature does suggest however that belief in personal control is associated with greater life-satisfaction, more positive self-concept and better emotional adjustment (Nehrke, Hulicka & Morganti, 1980; Palmore & Luikart, 1972; Wolk, 1976; Wolk & Kurtz, 1975). Wolk (1976) replicated previous research and found that internal locus of control was associated with positive self-concept, adjustment, satisfaction and higher activity levels among a group of elderly persons residing in a retirement village where few constraints were placed upon freedom of choice and where little emphasis was placed on engagement in structured organized activities. Reid et al. (1977) found that when locus of control is tied to more specific situations rather than general beliefs, the relationship between internality and self-concept and adjustment was much stronger. This would confirm the earlier differentiation made by Rotter (1966) about the relative role of specific and general expectancies. It suggests that locus of control may interact with situation-specific variables, and that an individual's perception of the linkage between personal effort and personal outcome depends a great deal upon the type of setting in which he is placed. Recently Wong and Sproule (1984) have contended that the majority of people, especially the elderly, embrace a dual-dimensional view of control. They have called them *bilocals*. Bilocals believe in the importance of both internal and external controls and do not regard these two types of controls necessarily inversely related as demanded by the unidimensional view.

Expanding on this idea, Kivett, Watson & Busch (1977) analyzed the relative importance of various physical, psychological and social variables in determining locus of control orientation in 337 adults aged forty-five to sixty-five. These authors found a strong relationship between internal locus of control and the nature of the individual's occupation, degree of religious motivation, and actual (as opposed to ideal) self-concept. As a possible mechanism for the increased risk of emotional problems and depression in older persons, this study suggests that the inevitable psychosocial losses and declines associated with aging may gradually erode healthy self-concept and self-esteem while the locus of control orientation simultaneously becomes more externally based.

Although the precise nature of the relationship between perceived locus of control and depression in older persons has yet to be elucidated fully, one plausible position is that locus of control is a rubric upon which the learned helplessness experimental analog of depression is directly based (Seligman, 1975; Maier & Seligman, 1976). Initially derived from experimental research with animals, the basic premise of learned helplessness is that the organism comes to perceive that personal responses have no effect in altering the environment. The typical learned helplessness paradigm involves animals that are subjected to an adverse situation which is not controllable, i.e., nothing the animal does in the attempt to extricate itself from the problem situation is successful. When confronted with such a set of contingencies, the animal quickly learns that avoidance is impossible and subsequently becomes "helpless." There is no further motivation and behavior takes on the appearance of apathy, resignation and helplessness. This reduced rate of response effort prevails even when the original contingencies are no longer operating, and this state of affairs is often labelled as part of the depressive's style of responding. Attempts to relate such conditions to clinical depression have not fared very well. This is discussed extensively in the special issue of *The Journal of Abnormal Psychology*, February, 1978.

However some attempts have been made to draw parallels with humans. Lewinsohn & Lee (1981) observed that depressed individuals perceive reinforcements as being basically unpredictable, outside their own control and dependent upon external factors such as chance, fate or powerful others. These authors maintained that the locus of control concept is a cognitive set that is subsumed by learned helplessness. Seligman (1975) argued that learned helplessness represented the clinical analog of depression and suggested that the attribution of external causality, i.e., the belief that outcomes are independent of responding, had motivational, cognitive and emotional consequences. This would account for the lowered rates of responding and reduced activity levels commonly associated with depression in all groups and particularly in the elderly. The cognitive distortion produced under such contingencies, i.e., rigidity, overgeneralization, magnification and pessimism about the future, is assumed to interfere with subsequent instrumental learning—which may explain the persistence of depression in many individuals. Finally, the emotional response of fear may be conceived as a stressor impinging upon the individual which sets into motion various biochemical, homeostatic mechanisms. These processes may initially be adaptive for the organism but are thought to break down when the stress experienced is of sufficient duration, as may be the case for chronic stress experienced by the elderly.

Locus of control therefore would seem to have particular importance in understanding the link between the cognitive and behavioral domains in mediation of depressive mood states. Furthermore, locus of control is especially applicable in any analysis of factors contributing to depression in the elderly. Research evidence has documented that advancing age nearly always involves the delegation of some authority and personal control as the individual relinquishes formerly held roles and increasingly relies upon external sources and significant others for essential needs (Brink, 1979; Butler & Lewis, 1973; Nehrke et al., 1980; Pfeiffer & Busse, 1973; Verwoerdt, 1976). Awareness of decreased personal control over outcomes often fosters the increased dependency seen in the elderly (Goldfarb, 1974), and this in turn can promote such depressive symptomatology as low rates of responsiveness, poor motivation, feelings of uselessness and hopelessness and lack of confidence.

Both Goldfarb (1974) and Brink (1979) have placed an emphasis on brief, problem-solving orientations in therapy with depressed older persons in which direct attempts to modify rigidity or change personal locus of control orientation are avoided. Instead, dependency and rigidity are recognized as potentially adaptive ego-defenses which may be used to encourage reliance and trust in the therapy. Thus, a potential liability may become an advantage in helping the older person deal with isolation, loneliness and despair.

PART TWO

PSYCHOTHERAPY STRATEGIES

CHAPTER V

RESEARCH IN GERIATRIC PSYCHOTHERAPY

Several comments regarding psychotherapy research in general and in specific relation to the elderly are indicated in order to provide a perspective for evaluating the available literature.

Current trends in psychotherapy process and outcome-research suggest that much progress has been achieved in pinpointing and ironing out methodological and theoretical problems with a corresponding increase in the level of precision afforded various therapy strategies (Phillips & Bierman, 1981). In particular, there have been notable advances in the assessment and treatment of depressed conditions based in part upon various cognitive and behavioral models of depression that stress the importance of a refined, empirical relationship between theory and therapy. Unfortunately, these encouraging developments, which testify to the burgeoning sophistication of contemporary psychotherapy research, have not been accompanied by similar advances in *geriatric* psychotherapy. For example, although Phillips & Bierman (1981) specifically reviewed the psychotherapy of depression, they did not report on any extension to elderly populations. Similarly, Lewinsohn & Lee (1981) noted a lack of systematic research devoted to the assessment and treatment of depression in the elderly.

The lack of a systematized body of research specifically focusing upon the application and utility of various therapy modalities with the elderly has been widely recognized (Gerner, 1979, Gottesman et al., 1973; Knight, 1979; Sparacino, 1979). This may stem, in part, from several factors. First, the scarcity of reports on psychotherapy with the elderly may reflect the perpetuation of a historical tendency to devalue or ignore the possibilities of conducting therapy with the elderly (Brink, 1979; Butler & Lewis, 1977; Ingebretson, 1977; Krasner, 1977; Rechtschaffen, 1959; Willner, 1978). A second reason may be the vigorous debate (Kastenbaum, 1978; Knight, 1979; Sparacino, 1979) about whether or not therapy techniques that have been used successfully with younger adults are just as readily applied to older adults. This uncertainty, coupled with prejudiced attitudes implying that change in older persons is unlikely, could help account for the relative lack of research in this area.

The point to be made here is simply that discussions and reports of principles of psychotherapy with the elderly essentially comprise the bulk of the available literature, and that the number of published therapy process or outcome-studies is so small as to be inconsequential. A further problem is the fact that most of these seminal discussions of psychotherapy techniques with the elderly stem from the traditional analytic-dynamic framework. Although they embody an elaborate, theoretically based rationale, these accounts are typically advanced without solid empirical support and typically include only case study reports which inevitably raise serious questions of reliability and generalization.

Given these problems and the paucity of research in psychotherapy with older persons in general, it should not be surprising that there is even less objective data specifically concerned with psychotherapy techniques for use with *depressed* elderly individuals. The next section reviews psychotherapy methods that have been incorporated for use with the elderly. Questions concerning the potential effectiveness of these methods in the treatment of depression and affective disorders in the elderly will then be addressed. Individual therapy strategies are discussed first, with the various theoretical orientations representing the continuum of therapy methods (i.e., insight-analytic, modified analytic, brief supportive therapy, cognitive behavioral) each being considered in turn. The latter part of this section will then focus upon group therapy.

CHAPTER VI

TRADITIONAL ANALYTIC THERAPIES

In a review of the literature on geriatric psychotherapy, Moss (1965) discriminatd between analytic therapies designed to facilitate insight and massive personality changes, and supportive analytic approaches aimed primarily at the alleviation of anxiety. Verwoerdt (1976) enumerated several distinctive features of insight-oriented therapy, including the use of free association and the analysis of the transference. The goal of insight-oriented therapy is not the solution of practical everyday problems but the alterations of personality structure so that the ego is gradually capable of assuming a more authoritative role in the intrapsychic life of the individual. The hallmark of this approach then, involves interpretation of unconscious maladaptive defenses and the restoration of the flexibility of the individual's character. Karpf (1977) differentiated between analytic and supportive psychotherapies noting that analysis involves making symptoms egoldystonic in order to permit insight and resolutions of unconscious conflicts, while supportive methods attempt to make symptoms ego-syntonic, less threatening and less likely to disrupt the equilibrium that the therapy seeks to restore.

The attempt to promote insight through interpretation and analogies of transference in therapy with older individuals has been questioned, however. As several writers (Karpf, 1977; Meerloo, 1955; Rechtschaffen, 1959; Verwoerdt, 1976) have suggested, the analysis of transference relationships in the elderly imposes special demands upon the therapist. Elderly patients may tend to unconsciously imbue the therapist with the characteristics of their children or grandchildren instead of viewing the therapist as a parent figure. Unless the therapist is experienced and aware of this symbolic relationship, the interpretations rendered may hinder rather than promote insight, complicating therapeutic progress (Butler & Lewis, 1977). Another problem for insight-oriented therapy is that frequently the elderly are more vulnerable to such explorations. Karpf (1977) indicated that because unconscious resistances and defenses may be weaker among the elderly, it may be easier to uncover elemental, primary process material which the individual is not adequately prepared to deal with. Therefore, the use of analytic techniques was advocated only with relatively intact, psychologically minded older persons whose level of emotional incapacitation was not severe.

Similarly, Brink (1979) in summarizing research, cast doubt upon the value of insight in psychotherapy with older persons, arguing that most of these patients lack the necessary ego-strength to capitalize on insight obtained in therapy. Fierman (1965) contended that insight could actually impede therapy by stimulating excessive rationalization and intellectualization as coping methods and promoting overt reliance upon these defense mechanisms. Thus, in immature or severely decompensated neurotic patients, insight may in fact reinforce neurotic tendencies. Wolberg (1943) maintained that delving into the genesis of maladaptive behavior, in essence, furnished an avoidance mechanism by which individuals could deny personal accountability for problems by attributing them to the influence of early life interpersonal relationships and environmental factors.

It has been extensively documented that the pioneer of psychoanalysis was not himself overly optimistic about the suitability of this approach as a treatment for the elderly (Brink, 1979; Cath, 1972; Freud, 1924; Knight, 1979; Rechtschaffen, 1959; Sparacino, 1979). Freud (1924) largely ignored personality changes associated with advanced age, viewing the psychopathology observed in later life as manifestations of unresolved early-life conflicts and traumas. Analytic therapy techniques were extensions of his theories of personality, psychosocial and sexual development which focused almost exclusively upon early childhood events (Brink, 1979). Freud (1924) believed that between the ages of forty-five and fifty, the individual began to lose the "elasticity of mental processes" characteristic of younger persons. As a result of age-related deterioration, it was felt that the individual gradually loses the ability to benefit from insight or cannot achieve insight at all. In contrast to later theorists who cautioned about the harmful effects of insight, Freud did not really consider the aged capable of responding to insight in the first place. He also believed that the analysis of older persons would be prolonged indefinitely by the sheer quantity of repressed material that it would be necessary to uncover in working back to early childhood, and that the elderly typically lacked the necessary motivation, stamina and patience required to deal with the demands imposed by analysis. Cath (1972) suggested however that Freud's earliest writings were unwarranted and premature extrapolations based upon his rather limited experiences with techniques which were themselves still in a state of evolution. Cath (1972) argued that towards the end of his life, Freud began to shift his earlier views concerning the potential for analytic therapy with older individuals, although he still maintained that such techniques were optimal with younger persons.

Whether ascribing to orthodox analytic methods or adhering to newer approaches that evolved from Freudian theory, subsequent analytic therapists were not as pessimistic as Freud. Abraham (1927, 1949), although in general agreement with Freud that the elderly are more rigid and less likely to successfully undergo massive personality reorganization, reported achieving success in psychoanalysis with persons older than fifty. He advocated an empirical approach in determining the parameters of effective therapy with older patients. One of the first successes was a case study of the analysis of a severely depressed fifty-year-old man who had required several hospitalizations. Specific details of treatment techniques were not elaborated

(Cath, 1972). On the basis of his own work, Abraham (1927) maintained that duration and severity of the disorder was a better predictor of therapy outcome than age per se. In other words, favorable prognosis was considered to be more a function of the recency of the acquired disorder than the age of the client. Abraham (1927) argued that it was possible to work back through the individual's life history if necessary but advocated treating reactive disorders of recent origin without a complicated and lengthy analysis. Implicit in this is the assumption that, for many persons, the emotional problems encountered in late life are reactive in nature, precipitated by unique stressors and accompanied by a steady decline from past levels of adaptation. Thus, Abraham (1927) was perhaps the first traditional dynamic analyst to suggest a more directive, active role for the therapist when treating the elderly.

Another early psychoanalyst who reported successful treatment with the elderly client was Jellifee (1925), who believed that aging was not necessarily a uniform process and that it did not necessarily produce qualitatively similar physiological or psychological changes in different individuals. Jellifee (1925) was decidedly conservative in his selection of appropriate candidates for analysis, and frequently refused treatment rather than modify his therapeutic method for those he considered unsuitable for analysis. This may have spuriously raised the number of treatment successes, and Jellifee himself maintained that the specific neurotic or psychotic symptoms exhibited by clients often represented better adaptive coping strategies than those that could be attained through intervention with psychoanalysis. Somewhat later, Fenichel (1945) took a similar position—that analysis is not effective in cases where the individual's physical and mental state is so impaired that it inhibits adoption of new coping strategies. Although he generally agreed with Freud's reservations regarding analysis with the elderly, Fenichel (1945) did suggest that analytic procedures could be applied to accomplish specific and immediate goals such as symptom removal (i.e., anxiety reduction) in lieu of achieving insight. In this way, Fenichel (1945) was somewhat more flexible than Jellifee (1925), and he anticipated the use of modified analytic techniques derived from the orthodox analytic framework.

A more encouraging outlook is apparent in the work of Kaufman (1937, 1940) who noted that conclusions concerning the inability of the elderly to achieve insight were subjective and not empirically derived. Kaufman (1940) reported several cases of successful analysis accompanied by fairly dramatic change in the condition of psychotically depressed individuals who were over age fifty-five. He disagreed with earlier ideas that analytic therapy with elderly patients necessitated extremely long periods of treatment before significant improvement could be detected. Unlike Freud, who thought that the ego gradually became rigid and unadaptive in old age, Kaufman (1940) interpreted rigidity as an ego-defense mechanism that could be ameliorated in therapy much as any other defensive maneuver. Thus, as Cath (1972) suggested, Kaufman was one of the first psychoanalysts to attempt analytic therapy with older persons without considering the age of the individual an obstacle to progress. The focus of therapy was not the restoration of the previous level of personality and emotional functioning, but rather the removal of symptoms and immediate resolution of problems.

For some 40 years following the intitial development

of psychoanalysis, within this movement very little attention was directed towards the goal of treating the emotional disorders of the aged, and even less was specifically focused upon analytic therapy of depression. The advent of Kaufman's (1937, 1940) published work with several depressed older persons represented a watershed that set the stage for subsequent modification and expansions of analytic methods for use with the elderly. Subsequently, the period from 1940-1960 was one of heightened interest in adapting psychoanalytic principles for the elderly. This renaissance was mainly due to an increased sense of optimism as the elderly were found to be capable of benefiting from therapy when appropriate modifications were introduced. The fact that modification of traditional analytic therapy was necessary only underscores more forcefully the impracticality of insight-oriented methods that did not concentrate on enabling the elderly to mobilize personal resources for solving immediate threats to physical and/or psychological well-being.

CHAPTER VII

MODIFIED ANALYTIC APPROACHES

The development of modified forms of therapy for use with the elderly has generally paralleled the evolution of theories of personality, which have increasingly attempted to address this group and incorporate aspects of the major task and goals confronting them. This precipitated a trend away from the psychoanalytic emphasis on the intense transference relationship and on resolution of intrapsychic conflicts towards more broadly scaled, environmentally oriented, and socially pragmatic interventions.

The steady growth of an ego psychology and ego-analytic orientation to therapies (Kastenbaum, 1978) is one example of this trend. White (1963) contended that the ego constituted the major vehicle for the control and direction of goal-directed behaviors. In this context, emotional disturbance in old age is viewed as a consequence of the breakdown of ego functions with a concomitant loss of self-esteem and sense of mastery and competence. This in turn interferes with the ability of the individual to cope with environmental change and tolerate new limitations of functioning imposed by physical changes. Brink (1979) argued for a more environmentally oriented therapy with the elderly— one that would be directed towards training them to substitute more adaptive behaviors and coping strategies as one means of facilitating a sense of achievement and mastery.

Alexander (1944) was one of the first analysts to modify psychoanalytic techniques to meet the needs of the elderly in therapy. He divided these modified techniques into insight-oriented versus supportive approaches, and drew a distinction between their primary treatment goals. Alexander (1944) defined insight therapy as the extension of ego control over previously repressed impulses, and argued that it would be unwise to attempt insight therapy in cases where the elderly person experienced a significant loss of ego strength. With these clients, Alexander (1944) advocated the use of a supportive therapy in which the therapist assumes a more directive role. Sparacino (1979) suggested that supportive techniques alleviated anxiety and inferiority feelings by providing reassurance and a permissive, protective relationship with the therapist. Karpf (1977) observed that supportive psychotherapy is the most commonly used form of individual treatment with older persons, and that it is effective across a wide range of both functional and organic disorders. He stressed that the main goal of such treatment is the facilitation of a sense of well-being, life satisfaction, and adjustment through the active cultivation of ego functioning. In this and other work (Alexander & French, 1946) however, depression was not specifically addressed in therapy. Nevertheless, Alexander's bifurcation of therapy strategy afforded a new flexibility by demonstrating that it was possible to alter traditional methodology with positive results. This in turn stimulated an increasing interest in further modifications of therapy both within and outside of the analytic framework.

One of the first cases in which modified analytic therapy was used to alleviate depression was reported by Gitelson (1948). The case involved a sixty-six-year-old depressed woman with insomnia, concentration difficulties and memory problems. Despite her husband's death six months previously, she could not express any overt signs of grief and complained of feeling empty and inadequate. The client had previously been in therapy with a different therapist, and Cath (1972) discussed the case in terms of the resolution of transference issues arising from this switch. He also noted that the therapy, involving twice weekly sessions over eight months, helped alleviate sexual inhibitions and guilt which were expressed in the form of conversion symptoms. The development of increased intrapersonal integration and capacity to relate to others was also reported.

Wayne (1953) advocated a modified analytic approach and suggested eight modifications of psychoanalysis appropriate to conducting therapy with the elderly. In this supportive approach, special emphasis was placed upon the solution of the client's most immediate problems. Probing to uncover older conflicts usually was not encouraged. The therapist reduced anxiety and dependency by formulating explicit goals and limitations of the therapy. The therapist assumed a fairly active role, and provided reassurance, guidance and environmental manipulations when appropriate. Wayne (1953) recommended that historical information be obtained to facilitate interpretations of tranference behaviors. Unlike early analytic therapy, this approach encouraged the client to sit facing the therapist to facilitate uncovering of repressed material. Perhaps the most fundamental departure from analytic methodology was the emphasis placed on the client's active participation in solving problems, and the minimization of the importance of insight. Discussion of cultural attitudes towards the elderly and the physiology of the aging process was encouraged to provide reassuring and normative feedback. He proposed that the duration of therapy be variable but generally time-limited, with from one to three sessions per week over a period of from six weeks to one year.

Wayne (1953) described a particular application of these techniques in the case of a sixty-six-year-old woman with depression stemming from the death of her mother. During the treatment, which lasted more than a year, this woman made significant progress in uncovering and more realistically handling repressed feelings—feelings that had been expressed as physical symptoms. Wayne (1953) concluded that therapy left the individual with better interpersonal skills and renewed capacity for work, and with amelioration of dysphoric mood. Again however, systematic, controlled, comparison outcome research was not attempted on the basis of clinical observations, and no objective measures of mood improvement were reported.

Other modified psychoanalytic strategies were advanced by Grotjahn (1955) and Meerloo (1955). These authors stressed the real and immediate needs of the client and how the therapist can fill the void created by the lack of significant interpersonal relationships. They also shared the view that the elderly often exhibit less resistance and react more favorably to interpretations and suggestions. Grotjahn (1955) elaborated three alternative responses to aging: normal integration and acceptance of life as it has been lived, increased rigidity and conservatism in trying to maintain defenses, and neurotic and/or psychotic regression.

Meerloo (1955, 1961) suggested that psychotherapy could be successful in up to half of all elderly cases. Rechtschaffen (1959) observed that Meerloo was in essential agreement with the view of other contemporary analytically oriented therapists. He emphasized the need for environmental modifications and the practice of "indeterminate termination" of clients. He advocated a gentle treatment of resistance and, like Grotjahn (1955), believed that with lessened resistance there is often a concomitant increase in access to the unconscious. Thus, Meerloo (1955) opposed the prevailing idea that the elderly were more rigid and therefore unsuitable for analytic treatment.

Weinberg (1951, 1975) also advocated an active, direct approach as a modification of analytic techniques. Weinberg (1975) stressed that the particular strategy used with older populations must always reflect their wide variability in physical condition, previous adaptation, degree of resistance to therapy, nature of transference, and history of symptomatology. General guidelines for therapy included the importance of empathy to encourage the open discussion of problems, relief of insecurity and anxiety, use of activities to increase self-esteem, and the use of community resources for the aged as an expression of concern and belief in the value and worth of the client. Weinberg (1957, 1970) stressed the need to consider factors such as life-style, previous adaptations, and present situation in therapy with the aged. He believed that therapy should be modified to deal with present problems instead of attempting to uncover the past, and suggested that therapy be of brief duration with frequent sessions.

Segal (1958) described a successful analysis using modified techniques. The patient was a seventy-three-year-old man who had remained in therapy for almost one and one-half years. This individual began therapy suffering from psychotic depression, paranoid delusions and rage attacks. After 18 months, a complete normalization of functioning was claimed. Segal (1958) hypothesized that the patient's breakdown was precipitated by an unconscious fear of death. Therapy centered upon overcoming the patient's use of denial and his over-idealized view of family members to facilitate expression of his anger and anxieties. Upon termination this patient reportedly drew closer to family members and was comforted by the realization that their lives would reflect family continuity even after his own death.

A somewhat different modification of therapy with the elderly is apparent in the work of Rockwell (1956), who advocated use of the Meyerian approach consisting of an analysis of all factors that could contribute to expression of symptoms. Thus, psychodynamic and somatic features as well as situational conditions and the constitutional make-up of the individual were considered. Each session was terminated with a constructive formulation and synopsis of material covered. This method was much more environmentally based and required the direct and active participation of both the therapist and *significant others* who assumed full responsibility for monitoring the patient's activities and collecting data based upon behavioral observations. Rockwell (1956) believed that therapy could precipitate anxiety reactions, somatic symptomatology, and depressions involving both fear and panic states. It was frequently observed that depression involved feelings of hopelessness and humiliation. The apathy engendered by these feelings was countered by an emphasis on work and structured activities aimed at overcoming progressive cycles of deterioration of functioning. Rechstschaffen (1959) criticized Rockwell's (1956) approach by suggesting that, although great emphasis was placed on understanding the total life situation of the patient, there was little practical application of this knowledge. In addition, no description of the general rationale underlying the management of the therapy itself was given. A further departure of this approach from analytic methods was the avoidance of repressed material. Free association was not encouraged because it was considered more beneficial to discuss neutral topics and thereby avoid contradictions and arguments.

By the 1960's the general consensus in psychoanalytic circles was that, in some cases, the elderly were capable of being helped in therapy. This period was marked by an increased awareness of the issues related to aging and depression and accompanied by an upsurge in publications (Berezin & Cath, 1965; Levin & Kahana, 1967; Zinberg & Kaufman, 1963). Levin (1965) focused upon depressive reactions in the elderly as a result of loss and disengagement. Levin (1963) argued that depression in the aged was reversible with therapy. He advocated activity and engagement rather than disengagement from the environment as a means of overcoming depressive mood. Levin (1965) proposed that the continuous accumulation of losses, with resulting disturbances of psychosocial equilibrium, constituted the basic source for the development of depression in older people. Emphasis in therapy was placed upon both internal and external factors and the importance of combating feelings of hopelessness and helplessness. Levin (1965) believed that in order to decrease the state of depression, the elderly must be given an opportunity to reinvest in satisfying object relationships that should allow them to develop some sense of hope and faith in the future.

Wolff (1963, 1970, 1971) reported a series of extensive, long-term therapy programs conducted with hospitalized, emotionally disturbed elderly patients as one example of the application of modified psychoanalytic approach involving both supportive and insight-oriented techniques. In his book on geriatric psychotherapy, Wolff (1970) described the treatment of a total of 54 elderly inpatients from various psychiatric facilities, manifesting both neurotic and psychotic symptoms. Although all patients were reportedly verbal and communicative, all demonstrated mild to moderate organic impairment. These individuals averaged nine years of hospital residency and were considered "hopeless" cases. Patients were tested both before and after initiation of psychotherapy, with a variety of depression measures, including the Wechsler-Bellevue, Rorschach and Thematic Apperception Test. Individual therapy sessions were conducted for 50 minutes per patient per week over a three month period.

The focus of therapy consisted of the attempt to

increase the patient's self-esteem through use of an ego-supportive technique. This involved reinforcing the individual's strengths. Wolff (1963, 1970) adopted the role of an empathetic, supportive "brother figure," and actively fostered hope and encouragement in patients. He encouraged them to openly discuss frustrations and ambivalent feelings resulting from their increased dependency. The goal of full insight was not a primary objective, although a limited form of insight was achieved by patients as a result of therapy, with the exception of the more severely regressed and withdrawn schizophrenic patients. According to Wolff (1963), full insight was prohibited due to an increased resistance and agitation encountered when the fear of death and dying was broached in therapy. Wolff (1963) suggested that such conflicts are more profitably left repressed.

With regard to outcome, Wolff (1963) reported that some improvement was noted in 34 of the 54 patients treated. One fourth of the patients demonstrated an increase in hostility towards the therapist and revealed increased anxiety as a function of treatment aimed at the attainment of partial insight. Three patients were classified as fully recovered although what this meant was not precisely defined. Twenty patients showed no improvement. Twenty-two of the 34 who improved were eventually discharged, although 12 of them were merely reassigned to various nursing or foster homes for continued care. Thus, discharge per se was not indicative of improvement or recovery. Interestingly, a one-year follow-up showed that all discharged patients had not needed rehospitalization and were maintaining satisfactory adjustment. Wolff (1970) noted that patients who left the hospital did so an average of four months following initiation of treatment; he took this to be encouraging in light of their lengthy period of hospitalization prior to treatment. It is also possible, however, that these individuals had not been as seriously ill as implied by their length of hospital residency.

Several criticisms of this program are possible. As with many other descriptions of therapy interventions with the elderly, outcome measures lacked precision and comparability across various treatment groups. Although Wolff (1970) was careful to establish drug-only and milieu-therapy control groups, comments on outcome were restricted to subjective evaluations of improvement. Relevant data concerning cognitive functioning or changes in projective and intellectual test instruments were omitted. Another significant problem with this project was the failure to render the therapist blind regarding classification of patients as members of particular treatment groups. Finally, Wolff (1963, 1970) did not incorporate a no-treatment control group in order to eliminate non-specific factors as an explanation for results obtained. Despite these shortcomings, the contributions of Wolff's (1970) research did have a significant impact in shaping more positive attitudes among providers of mental health care to residential elderly populations.

In later research, Wolff (1971) continued to use a modified psychoanalytic approach in specifically addressing the treatment of the depressed and suicidal geriatric patient. He argued that such treatment required understanding of the sources of the patient's depressions. In order to accomplish this, the therapist must consider the individual's personality, family situation, and other environmental influences, including the immediate stressors, which may have precipitated the depression. Wolff (1971) cautioned that, unless a broad understanding of these factors is achieved, the treatment of depression and suicidal tendencies becomes overly simplistic and leads to the complacent misuse and excessive reliance on antidepressant drugs or electroconvulsive therapy.

Wolff (1971) categorized two hundred male geriatric patients on the basis of the above criteria and involved two groups of one hundred individuals each. Both groups consisted of patients with current and previous histories of depression but were divided into suicidal and non-suicidal groups. In the non-suicidal group (Group A) the symptoms of depression were related to the issue of loss or failure, while in Group B symptoms of depression were related psychodynamically to compulsivity. Group A patients exhibited psychomotor retardation in speech and thought, anorexia or weight gain, insomnia and restlessness. They felt useless and worthless and without significant goals in life or a plan for the future. They had numerous somatic complaints as well. Their basic personality structure was described as passive-dependent in nature, characterized by emotional immaturity and oral tendencies such as strong desires for acceptance and sympathy. By contrast, Group B individuals expressed more irritability, hostility, and agitation and expressed them more frequently and intensely than Group A individuals.

Wolff (1971) interpreted these differences with psychodynamic language and constructs. He believed that the depressions of Group A individuals represented a typical pattern in response to loss of such things as physical health, social status, relatives and friends, or of independence and financial security. He classified the majority of these patients as either psychosomatic or psychoneurotic. The more seriously depressed patients of Group B represented a life pattern based on hard work, compulsive striving for achievement and perfection, and were perceived as generally more inflexible and more resistant to changed circumstances or environments. The majority of these individuals were diagnosed as having psychotic depressive reactions.

Wolff (1971) proceeded to draw distinctions between the psychotherapies appropriate to each of the groups, based upon inferences concerning their basic personality differences. Severely depressed, suicidal patients with overly rigid superego controls, introjected hostility, and compulsiveness necessitated firmness and a critical attitude on the part of the therapist. The passive dependent elderly individual with neurotic characteristics responded more favorably however when empathetic understanding and genuine kindness were employed in therapy. Wolff (1971) suggested that these individuals responded rather well to individual psychotherapy and reported success with 22 patients where individual therapy involving fifty-minute sessions on a weekly basis over a three to six month period was the focus of treatment. This group of patients had low self-esteem, and manifested dependency feelings about being superfluous, rejected and unwanted. Loss was an important dynamic underlying depression in this group. Wolff (1971) emphasized the importance of helping the patient rediscover former hobbies and interests that could become an alternative career. This aspect of therapy was credited with imparting a new sense of purpose and encouragement to many individuals. Wolff (1971) credited the opportunity to meet new people, develop new friendships and engage in new activities, with being crucial in overcoming isolation, low self-esteem and feelings of inadequacy. He concluded that, with these depressed elderly persons, the therapist should assume a supportive role and that treatment usually ought to be on an out-patient basis.

The therapist is advised in these cases to avoid adoption of an authoritative, strict or punishing stance.

Quite a different picture is presented for the therapy of suicidal, depressed geriatric patients. Wolff (1971) maintained that the goal of treatment for these individuals should be decreased hostility through sublimation of anger into constructive activities. The issue of control is important, and the therapist is advised to maintain a more demanding, authoritative profile. Wolff (1971) suggested that, although individual and group psychotherapy may facilitate verbalization of hostility, the use of both antidepressant and electroconvulsive techniques may be required when the danger of suicide is imminent. Wolff (1971) noted that careful monitoring of these individuals was mandatory and that electroconvulsive therapy often constituted a more effective treatment in terms of response time. Wolff (1971) observed that the treatment of depressed older persons is enhanced when treatment is based upon analyses of dynamic features, thus implying that proper evaluation and diagnosis are a prerequisite for appropriate interventions. This may seem obvious, but particularly in medical practice, treatment is often undertaken without precise diagnosis.

The rationale underlying Wolff's (1971) research is essentially the same philosophy presented by Willner (1978). In this view, the treatment of depression in the elderly would be enhanced if different diagnostic categories of depression could be identified along with the specific modalities of psychotherapy that are most appropriate. Willner (1978) reported the use of insight oriented, psychodynamically based psychotherapy over a three-year period at an outpatient clinic along with some preliminary outcome evaluations of this program. Results of this treatment modality appeared to have been generally positive, with Willner (1978) indicating that most elderly, depressed outpatients did benefit from psychotherapy. Willner (1978) stated that additional research was currently in progress to determine relative effectiveness of specific treatment parameters (i.e., individual versus group, insight-oriented versus supportive) in therapy with elderly depressed patients. This work should shed further light on the utility of various therapy modalities and perhaps lend support to the typology proposed above by Wolff (1971).

All of the therapies discussed above attempt to utilize insight, in varying degrees, as a curative technique. It should be apparent, however, that the term itself may connote different meanings to different therapists and that insight therapy with the elderly does not necessarily embody or typify the classic, orthodox analytic concept of insight. Similarly, the use of insight does not necessarily constitute an endorsement of the classic analytic approach. To illustrate this point, supportive, analytically oriented therapies which have de-emphasized the role of insight are discussed below.

The views of Pfeiffer (1971), along with Busse (Busse & Pfeiffer, 1973) accelerated the shift towards a more supportive style of therapy with older persons. Pfeiffer (1971) presented an outline of revisions of traditional psychotherapy which were based upon Rogerian concepts of unconditional acceptance, warmth and genuineness. Busse & Pfeiffer (1973) believed that substantial modifications of traditional analytic therapy were necessary in order for therapy to be practical with the majority of older persons. They stressed the need for increased therapist initiative in probing to identify areas of conflict, in establishing immediate, specific therapy goals, and in using "symbolic giving" (i.e., the creation by the therapist of a warm and friendly atmosphere) to partially compensate for the client's social and physical losses. The importance of therapist empathy and identification with the client was underscored, and the need to be aware of the special nature of transference and countertransference problems was stressed. The limited goals of therapy were defined as symptom relief, support for new adaptation to changes in life-styles, acceptance of increased dependency as a natural by-product of the aging process, and the prescription for continued or renewed involvement in a variety of activities. In his work, Pfeiffer (1971) noted that the elderly are typically highly responsive to therapy and concluded that, in terms of the investment of time, outcome of therapy is often more dramatic with older than with younger individuals.

Verwoerdt (1976) has presented techniques constituting a psychodynamically oriented, supportive therapy with elderly clients. Regression and transference issues are de-emphasized and not interpreted. The goal of facilitating insight is replaced by the attempt to shore up existing coping mechanisms in order to enhance the individual's ability to overcome current hardships. This supportive approach attempts to discover and strengthen adaptive defenses, and the client is encouraged to substitute these for maladaptive ones. The goal of therapy is restabilization and the client's return to a more satisfactory level of equilibrium. Verwoerdt (1976) discussed the relationship aspects of pyschotherapy as a form of both communication and metacommunication. He emphasized the need to monitor nonverbal communication to avoid sending the implicit message that the client is unimportant. Verwoerdt (1976) maintained that therapy should reflect an atmosphere of detached concern and represent a balance between gentleness and firmness. He stressed the desirability of fostering hope, and security and the preservation of dignity. Other important aspects of therapy were the ability to provide calm and sincere reassurance, emphasizing the positive strengths of the client, and strengthening the client's sense of personal identity by promoting a sense of control, mastery and effectiveness. It is interesting to note that these latter ideas incorporate recent variables thought to be key components in the process leading to depression and other forms of psychopathology (Bandura, 1977).

Grigorian (1970) advocated an empathetic, supportive approach in the treatment of depressed older persons based upon the assumption that depression in late life is due to unsuccessful adaptation to losses. He noted that losses were a quantitative function of age, with losses increasing in direct proportion to longevity. Grigorian (1970) stressed direct observation of behavior and appearance, obtaining of a detailed life-history to determine qualitative and quantitative parameters of losses experienced, and the expression of empathy and warmth along with hope and reassurance.

Grigorian (1970) discussed the treatment of a sixty-nine-year-old married woman who had experienced a depression of six months duration consisting of periods of sadness, crying spells, frequent somatic complaints, and concentration difficulties. An initial physical examination revealed no organic basis for the woman's abdominal pain, and a complete history revealed that the patient had had two prior episodes of depression, at age thirty and fifty-two. Both were accompanied by symptoms such as psychomotor retardation, exhaustion, insomnia, anorexia, and weight loss. These symptoms had responded well to psychotherapy. On initial interview for the current depressive episode, the patient was agitated, tearful, and expressed feelings of helplessness. Psychotherapy was again initiated and was continued on a weekly basis over a nine month period. These sessions revealed that, just prior to onset of her depression, a young student who had boarded with the patient and her husband for two years had left. The woman, who was childless, had felt a strong attachment to the student and expressed the wish that he were her own son. This woman also discussed her anxiety regarding her future and her physical health. She was angry and concerned about her husband's perceived lack of sympathy, and about his inability to care for her if she became ill. A mild stroke the previous year had left him incapacitated. In the course of therapy, Grigorian (1970) reported that this woman was helped to adjust to the loss of the "surrogate child" by focusing on an analysis of the symbolic meaning the young man had acquired in her life. The threat posed to the woman by the loss of youth, and age-related decline in physical functioning was also a major focus of therapy. In time, the patient began to integrate her perceptions of her role as an older woman more realistically. She adjusted to the social limitations imposed by the aging process. This improved her self-image and self-esteem and facilitated more adaptive, healthy ego-functioning.

The use of supportive, modified analytic psychotherapy is also reported in several case reports. Zarsky & Blau (1970) discussed the treatment of regression and dependency in a sixty-year-old woman who remained in treatment sporadically over a period of ten years. Hauser (1968) commented on psychotherapeutic intervention with a seventy-eight-year-old depressed woman who had totally denied all aspects of her aging.

This individual had experienced an initial severe depressive breakdown at age fifty which responded to electroconvulsive therapy and supportive psychotherapy. Hauser (1968) used a supportive approach to help the woman acknowledge fears of aging and death and reported some symptomatic improvement over a period of several months. Da Silva (1967) presented the case of an eighty-one-year-old, lonely, depressed man who had been hospitalized several times previously, beginning at age eighteen. In the course of three years at a state hospital, psychotherapy was reportedly able to facilitate some insight and instill hope. The supportive framework also provided reassurance which reduced anxiety and withdrawal.

Wasser (1966) discussed the relevance of Hartmann's (1958) model of emotional adaptation of the elderly and the aging process. She stressed the importance of a thorough diagnostic evaluation of the aged person that emphasized knowledge of family and personal history, typical response styles and developmental tasks and past crises, as well as an estimation of present capacity for social functioning. Wasser (1966) favored the use of supportive therapy with older persons and believed that such techniques increased capacity for self-mobilization through the simultaneous relief of internal and external stress and the strengthening of useful defenses.

Feigenbaum (1974) argued that depression should be viewed as the major emotional illness or problem of aged persons. He pointed out that drug and sexual problems in the elderly pose significant complications in the management and process of psychotherapy. The use of drugs given for symptomatic relief of problems (such as insomnia), which often are direct manifestations of depression, may actually exacerbate the primary problem of dysphoric mood. Sexual problems also complicate therapy for depression because the patient's anxiety about diminished sexual capacity often contributes markedly to decreased self-esteem. According to Feigenbaum (1974), depression is frequently precipitated by interpsychic problems stemming from loss of physical, social, economic and emotional supports. Thus, Feigenbaum (1974) agreed with the idea previously outlined that loss is related to the development of depression, although he was quick to point out that the elderly do not necessarily experience depression in any qualitatively different fashion than younger persons. He argued that the lack of gerontologic education and countertransference feelings on the part of the therapist frequently constituted an external factor that complicated the emotional problems of the elderly. Feigenbaum (1974) was aware of the importance of careful deliberation concerning appropriate treatment goals and strongly believed that improvement rates of the elderly in psychotherapy were comparable to those attained by younger age groups.

Safirstein (1972) was another therapist who advocated a psychodynamic point of view in a functional approach to the treatment of mental illness in the elderly. The goal of therapy was to help the individual reestablish premorbid levels of functioning as much as possible in order to prolong maintenance within the community and postpone or totally obviate the need for institutionalization. Although Safirstein (1972) did not regard long-term therapy as mandatory, he conceded that it was sometimes called for in order to stabilize and support an individual's functioning within the community when the alternative would be institutionalization. (When institutionalization does not take place, the link with the community is not always present. The best examples are the homeless mentally ill of today.) Safirstein (1972) asserted that the objective of therapy was to foster independence in the elderly through use of their existing assets and resources. He believed that this was feasible in spite of their tendency towards decreased flexibility and impaired adaptive capacity.

Safirstein (1972) regarded depression in the elderly as a frequent concomitant of the unravelling of the individual's social, environmental and physical status quo. Depressive mood was held to be a reaction to disruptions in the person's capacity to tolerate changes in equilibrium. Safirstein (1972) noted that depressed older persons often had been depressed earlier in life but, because they had more adequate resources available to them, they did not require help to the same degree as when older. Similar to analytic and ego-analytic theorists (Freud, 1924; Levin, 1965), Safirstein (1972) hypothesized that the crucial issue in the depressions of older persons was their increased vulnerability to losses in all spheres due to aging. Safirstein (1972) noted that psychotherapy with older, depressed persons was rewarding and that, even if lengthier therapy was necessary to provide long-term support, therapeutic results were often dramatic. Although he reported being able to conclusively terminate treatment for about 70 percent of his clients, Safirstein (1972) observed that it was common for treatment to be reinstated later on with the focus on another problem. The underlying assumption was that old age is a chronic condition with increased probability for some type of emotional disequilibrium requiring therapeutic intervention.

In stressing the vitality of supportive therapy in the treatment of depression, Neumann (1974) noted the critical importance of somatic symptoms as expressions of underlying depression. He regarded somatic problems as perhaps the cardinal sign of depression among the elderly. Somewhat in congruence with dynamic theories of the etiology of depression, Neumann (1974) believed there was almost always an identifiable triggering mechanism to explain the onset of depression. This could be a developmental or life-history milestone such as retirement, stress associated with the loss of a spouse, or adjustment to a sudden, incapacitating physical illness. Again, all of these factors can be distilled into a form of loss or threat to the individual's ability to cope, adjust and integrate change. Neumann (1974) hypothesized that depression in the elderly represented the individual's responses to unpleasant external realities. He observed several prominent behavioral manifestations of depression including early morning awakenings, hopelessness, anxiety, and excessive guilt, pity and self-concern. As Verwoerdt (1976) might hypothesize, these response styles in turn could further erode the *capacity* of the elderly to make use of their internal and external environmental experiences for coping and mastery. This illustrates the interacting effect of internal capacity and external stress. Personal ineffectiveness (Bandura, 1977; Beck, 1976), negative cognitive distortions and sense of personal helplessness (Seligman, 1975) have all been implicated as fostering dysphoric mood states and will be discussed below in connection with behaviorally oriented therapy.

Although Neumann (1974) regarded the judicious use of antidepressant medication as warranted, he was also in essential agreement with the position later taken by Karpf (1980) that medication alone was rarely helpful without some kind of supportive therapy. In Neumann's (1974) view, medication in combination with therapy was effective in ameliorating the depressions of elderly patients within six weeks in about half of all cases. Neumann's (1974) approach exhibited an awareness that supportive psychotherapy can play a useful role in alleviating depression through establishment of concrete, pragmatic and stable therapeutic relationships. In the final analysis, the relative utility of medication versus psychological therapies may have to be judged by comparing such variables as cost-effectiveness and response time and by calculating the severity of the depression. It is perhaps mainly for this reason that it has become increasingly popular to consider the advantages of briefer duration psychotherapy.

CHAPTER VIII

BRIEF PSYCHOTHERAPY

Although largely based on psychoanalytic concepts, the brief psychotherapy approach as pioneered by Goldfarb (1955, 1956) created a dramatic shift in the focus of psychotherapy with geriatric populations. As Brink (1979) observed, this modality and other modifications based on it, such as the problem-solving orientations, have become the treatment of choice for working with elderly clients. As early as 1953, Havinghurst and Albrecht had recommended informal counseling and training in coping skills for the elderly. From this Goldfarb (1956) argued that the rationale for psychotherapy with the elderly should be based on the assumption that their behavior was goal-directed and oriented towards problem-solving. Other therapists (Bennett, 1973; Safirstein, 1972; Seegal, 1956) echoed this view. Safirstein (1972) believed the therapist should intervene quickly and decisively and then fade out as the crisis recedes. Earlier Seegal (1956) articulated a "principle of minimal interference" which held that the older the patient, the less one should disturb established patterns of living.

The major feature of Goldfarb's (1955, 1956) brief psychotherapy was the deliberate attempt to use the increased dependency of the elderly as a therapeutic resource. Futhermore, depression was acknowledged as the central factor motivating the elderly to seek treatment, and depression was considered the integral theme underlying the expression of symptoms. Feelings of hopelessness and helplessness were considered pervasive in old age and were traced to the existence of these factors during earlier years. Goldfarb (1955, 1956) postulated that dependency and helplessness were basic motivational forces for most individuals in our culture, and were therefore adaptive forces in the elderly. Indeed, it was assumed that attempts to avoid the dependency issue in therapy with older persons would paradoxically lead to a therapist-patient struggle that would inevitably result in an increased sense of inadequacy and helplessness in the patient. Goldfarb (1955, 1956) argued that acceptance of the dependencies of the older patient could be used in therapy to instruct and encourage more efficient, acceptable, adaptive behavior patterns. In this approach, the therapist was advised to adopt a reassuring, supportive, goal-directed method of interacting with elderly patients. The therapist therefore must not attempt to dispel the image or role model of surrogate parent that he acquires in the course of therapy.

While depression is viewed as a cardinal feature to be dealt with in therapy with the elderly, the major feature of Goldfarb's (1955, 1956) brief psychotherapy was the deliberate attempt to use the increased dependency as a therapeutic resource. Goldfarb (1955, 1956) attempted to maximize a process of reversed transference whereby the therapist is embued with parental attributes by the client and is perceived as an almost omnipotent figure. Through this relationship, Goldfarb (1955, 1956) argued that gratification of emotional needs to be met and feelings of fear, anger, tension and anxiety could be dispelled. A major advantage of specifically addressing and working with the increased dependency of the elderly is that the therapy does not require a great many creative emotional resources within the client. The therapy is conducted on a simple relationship level so that there is little demand for the intellectual capabilities required by insight and introspective methods. This approach originated within an institutionalized setting where many individuals suffered from chronic organic brain syndromes. Problems arising from defensive resistance and rigidity are side-stepped because there is no emphasis on a dramatic restructuring of personality. Goldfarb (1955, 1956) reported that brief therapy was much more efficient and cost-effective and often was successful with less than 15 minutes of patient contact per week.

Goldfarb's brief therapy has been criticized on several fundamental points (Brink, 1979; Knight, 1979; Sparacino, 1979). One problem in cultivating a dependent relationship to such a high degree is the risk that patients may quite readily relapse without continuous contact with the therapist. This issue has not been fully explored, although it seems likely that all patients, especially more regressed individuals, may evidence increased instability and adjustment difficulties upon loss of the significant relationship represented by one's therapist. Conceivably, many personality and environmental factors may play a role in determining both the scope of the dependency and the reaction to termination of treatment. The therapist should certainly consider these factors prior to the termination of treatment. Another criticism has been that the practical application of this type of therapy may be restricted to institutional settings where the control by the therapist is more complete. Finally, the practice of encouraging illusions in patients regarding the omnipotence of the therapist, when realistic alternative solutions are available, is questionable from an ethical standpoint. Regrettably, little in the way of empirical validation of Goldfarb's technique has subsequently appeared in the literature (Sparacino, 1979). Despite these problems and criticisms, however, Kastenbaum (1978) argued that these brief-therapy procedures constitute a valuable means of helping people who manifest significant psychological and organic impairments who might otherwise not be considered amenable to therapy.

Additional support for the use of brief psychotherapy with elderly patients was provided by Bennett (1973) who found that short-term psychotherapy and dependency on the authority of others were the primary ingredients in the treatment of the aged, depressed psychiatric patient. This approach also was deemed more appropriate with more severely depressed, hospitalized individuals. Safirstein (1972) recommended the use of brief therapy with a psychodynamic orientation to focus upon a specific, immediate problem requiring decisive, immediate intervention and a quick retreat by the therapist.

Several case studies employing brief therapy have demonstrated the effectiveness of this technique. Hammer (1972) discussed the case of a sixty-eight-year-old man who played piano professionally and who suffered depression related to the loss of his musical abilities due to failing eyesight and chronic arthritis. This had resulted not only in the loss of a meaningful activity but precipitated considerable reduction of self-esteem and sense of fulfillment. Depression was exacerbated by persistent confusion about his identity and purpose and by additional aversive consequences resulting from the loss of his source of livelihood and the recent death of his wife. The patient perceived himself bereft of the support provided by spouse, friends, children, career and good physical health. In the initial stages of treatment, the patient revealed many chronic, maladaptive personality deficits such as dependency, inability to make friends, inferiority feelings and excessive fear of dying. The goals of therapy were to overcome his tendency to concentrate upon the past and to instill hope that the future could be promising. Other vocational possibilities were explored, and the therapist assisted the patient in locating a job as a piano teacher. This remotivated the patient and provided him with a new source of income, personal status, human contact and an outlet for artistic expression. Hammer (1972) reported that by the sixth session the patient no longer ruminated about past injustices, the death of his wife, current difficulties or fear of death. At this point, the patient terminated futher treatment concluding that he would not require further assistance.

Blau & Berezin (1975) discussed a case involving a

seventy-five-year-old man who exhibited intense anxiety and depression related to a fear of dying of cancer. The client viewed some of his symptoms as similar to those exhibited by an older brother who had recently died and left his younger sibling feeling vulnerable. Rather than embarking upon a lengthy analysis of the client's sibling relationships, the therapist arranged for the client to move in with a younger relative who could assume a protective role similar to the one once played by the older brother. After a total of four sessions, this intervention had resulted in a considerable reduction in the client's anxiety and depressed mood.

Brink (1977) discussed tenets of brief psychotherapy and illustrated its use with a case history involving a suicidal, sixty-four-year-old woman who complained of insomnia and feelings of uselessness, helplessness and emptiness. Therapy was time-limited of necessity as the woman was seen while the therapist was on a 15-day trip in a foreign country. According to Brink (1977) this client had a long history of self-punishing behaviors and psychosomatic disturbances. These were aggravated by the recent death of her husband and eldest son. The most recent precipitating event had been the decision of her thirty-four-year-old daughter to marry and move to another city. Therapy focused upon the woman's active problem-solving abilities rather than an analysis of the repetitious and self-defeating tendency to inflict self-punishment through physical channels. The client had been active and showed no organic impairment or chronic physical illness. She wanted to continue to live in her large home and run it as a boarding house for medical students, but her family disapproved of this plan. The therapist helped to implement this plan by convincing family members of its value in contributing to alleviation of the client's depression. No antidepressant medication or electroconvulsive therapy was employed and the client, a religious woman, was encouraged to continue her prayer as a means of disrupting suicidal ideas. Treatment consisted of four hour-long sessions over a 15-day period, and brought about a lifting of dysphoric mood and lessening of psychosomatic complaints. Unfortunately, due to the nature of the therapeutic arrangement no follow-up data was provided to monitor stability and duration of behavioral improvement.

Brink's (1977, 1979) approach to brief therapy diverged from that of Goldfarb (1955, 1956). He argued that brief therapy is primarily designed to help the individual cope with problems unique to the latter part of life such as retirement, widowhood, chronic physical problems and changed living arrangements. The therapist must not only be an empathetic listener, but must also be able to promote the restructuring of the client's interactions within the environment. In Brink's (1977) review, brief therapy does not require a focus upon transference and dependency issues. Goldfarb (1956), however, contended that dependency may be capitalized on and manipulated therapeutically within the context of transference and that transference issues do not dissolve merely because the therapist pretends to ignore them. Based upon research (Lipman & Smith, 1968; Palmore, 1968) demonstrating that depression is less likely when the elderly individual is more active, Brink (1977) concluded that brief therapy for depression should be primarily supportive and should encourage activity rather than introspection. Although longer-term therapy might more easily facilitate intrapsychic processes such as the redirecting of anger, the time-limited format advocated by Brink (1977, 1979) concentrated instead upon efforts to increase activation and participation in the environment. To be effective in this regard, the therapist must assume the role of social planner, family counselor, mediator, and rehabilitator. The formation of classic transference is side-stepped in favor of enlisting the patient's cooperation in finding useful solutions to problems. Brink (1977) noted that mild depression constitutes the major psychiatric problem of the elderly, and that inferiority feelings rather than guilt tend to predominate as precipitating factors. Nevertheless, Brink (1977) argued that depression often increases suicide risk, and he suggested that the goal of reducing suicidal feelings is obviously best realized through control of the depression which precipitated them. Brief therapy accomplishes this by activating the patient and engaging and utilizing those abilities, interests or skills available and well-established in the client. For example, in the case described above, Brink (1977) capitalized on the client's religious devotion by encouraging her to use prayer as a means of interrupting suicidal rumination.

The main difference between brief therapy and longer-term therapy is that brief therapy tends to be more environmentally oriented and supportive. It generally seeks to elicit the active participation and cooperation of the client and sets attainable goals to facilitate rapid change. The importance of insight and transference is minimized, although some intuitive awareness on the part of the individual is certainly useful to the therapist. Thus, brief therapy has emerged as a pragmatic, problem-solving orientation mirroring the prevailing trend towards streamlining the therapy process. Brief psychotherapy with a problem-solving orientation thus helps the individual to define problems, collect facts, generate workable solutions, narrow down and select the most efficacious course of action, and then implement the plan. This procedure of testing hypotheses is then subject to continual modification based upon feedback and evaluation of results. The concern of the therapist is with here-and-now problems; introspection, concern about the past, and anxiety about the future is de-emphasized. The therapist should take an active role fulfilling the multiple roles of social planner, vocational consultant and rehabilitator, and family counselor (Zinberg, 1967). Transference and dependency issues are usually avoided in this form of brief therapy (Safirstein, 1972), although, as noted above, analytically oriented brief therapy (Goldfarb, 1956) will typically address these issues in working with clients.

All of the case reports discussed above incorporate problem-solving methodology in the treatment of depression with brief therapy. Some controlled, comparative-outcome research data using brief problem-solving therapy with the elderly has been reported (Garner & Korzeniowski, 1971; Godbole & Verinis, 1974; Lazarus & Fay, 1975). However, methodological weaknesses have limited their usefulness. In one such comparative study, Godbole & Verinis (1974) explored the effectiveness of brief psychotherapy with physically ill, elderly patients. Their rationale for using this type population was that, since psychological problems may interfere with medical treatment complicating recovery, psychotherapy should be incorporated as part of any comprehensive treatment package. Inpatients suffering from incapacitating illness (i.e., heart disease) were assigned to one of three conditions. One group received brief supportive therapy, while a second group received a brief problem-solving method via the use of a confrontation statement. This involved presenting the patients with direct confrontation statements challenging the beliefs and fears that were associated with their central conflicts and which resulted in maladaptive behavior patterns. Both therapy groups received between 6 and 12 therapy sessions three times weekly for 10 to 15 minutes. A control group received only two evaluation interviews and did not participate in therapy. Dependent measures involved objective and subjective rating scales filled out by the therapist and medical personnel concerning various areas of the patient's functioning including depression, insomnia, and anxiety. In addition, self-report measures of self-concept and depression were obtained, as well as indices concerning discharge plans and anticipated progress or rehabilitation. Relative efficacy of the three treatment conditions was assessed through analysis of pre-post difference scores on these measures. Results showed that the confrontation group exhibited significantly more postitive changes overall than the non-confrontation and control groups for both therapist and nurse-rated variables. Futhermore, only the confrontation group demonstrated a significant improvement on measures of depression and self-concept.

This study suffered from several methodological problems that raise serious questions about the validity of the results. For example, the raters were not blind with respect to subjects' membership in a particular treatment condition. Furthermore, the therapist conducting treatment was under the direct supervision of the originator of the confrontation technique which raises the possibility that experimenter expectancies and bias inflated ratings of success on depression measures for the confrontation therapy group. An additional problem was the failure to employ adequate statistical controls, such as analysis of covariance for the control condition, in which significant relationships were found between improvement in depression and self-concept, and extraneous factors such as marital status and use of psychotropic medication. In spite of these difficulties, this study does suggest that use of stepwise problem-solving techniques in brief therapy can lead to reduced depression in elderly hospitalized persons. Future research should address these problems through incorporation of appropriate methodological refinements that will permit more unambiguous interpretation of results.

Behaviorally oriented treatment approaches—which are themselves generally philosophically committed towards short-term intervention and the active, directive participation of the therapist in the management of therapy—may overlap to a great extent with other problem-solving and supportive, brief-therapy methods. Before turning to an examination of these treatment strategies, however, it would be a serious omission not to scrutinize what has been termed one of the most significant and widely employed psychotherapy techniques in treating the elderly (Brink, 1979): the life review. Life review therapy was first proposed by Butler (1964) and subsequently expanded by Lewis & Butler (1974). In this procedure, the therapist assumes an active, directing role facilitating a detailed reconstruction of the individual's history and accomplishments. Lewis & Butler (1974) described the use of various methods of aiding the process of efficient and deliberate recollection of life events including compilation of photo albums, scrapbooks, and other personal records. Reunions, visits to previously important places and reconstruction of family history and genealogy are also important. The life review process is meant to help reconstruct the elderly client's sense of identity, allow acceptance of past failures, and bring about a fuller understanding of personal limitations. This

technique is somewhat loosely based upon free association and does require an alert, verbal and motivated
client with fairly intact ego-defenses. Therefore, to the
extent that the client is incapacitated by severe neurotic conflicts or major depressive illness, this technique may be contraindicated (Brink, 1979).

Despite these limitations, Lewis & Butler (1974)
maintained that the elderly often spontaneously review
their lives in an existential drive to seek meaning, solve
problems and achieve emotional gratification. Lewis &
Butler (1974) strongly advocated the use of individual
psychotherapy in any encounter with the elderly, and
they indicated that the presence of organic impairment
does not necessarily exclude positive gains. They contended that the elderly seek to verbalize their experiences and escape boredom and often quite naturally focus
upon present rather than future concerns as a direct
result of an acute awareness of the passage of time.
This process shares many of the features embodied by
a supportive therapy approach. The life review process
can also be useful in confronting conflicts and anxiety
concerning the inevitability of death. Themes of guilt
and restitution often figure prominently in life review
therapy as existential concerns are magnified. The life
review process seems to partially confirm Erikson's
(1968) life span personality development model, which
postulated that older individuals are often motivated
by the need to develop a sense of their own position and
contribution relative to past and present generations
in order to place their lives in perspective.

Compared with more analytically oriented brief
therapies, it is considered more important in life review
techniques to help the elderly continue to confront
problem areas. The value or necessity of "curing" the
individual is de-emphasized. Unlike Goldfarb's (1955,

1956) approach, Lewis & Butler (1974) presumed the need for an active rather than passive-dependent patient role in therapy. They have also suggested the use of various self-confrontational techniques in the life review process. In contrast to this philosophy, Pitt (1974) argued that dynamic considerations do not lose significance in the elderly and that it is still important to address intrapsychic as well as interpersonal conflicts. Thus, Pitt (1974) adopted a stance more in line with Goldfarb (1955, 1956) in suggesting the establishment of a supportive relationship to satisfy dependency needs. Like Lewis & Butler (1974), however, Pitt (1974) recognized the value of getting the elderly patient to consolidate experiences using reminiscence as a device for eliminating repetitive complaints and promoting conflict resolution. Blau & Berezin (1975) also emphasized the usefulness of reminiscences about earlier accomplishments and gratifications as a means of fostering self-esteem. In spite of the widespread popularity of the process of life review as a therapy with the elderly, surprisingly little research has directly examined its use in the treatment of depression. It is lamentable that, to date, no well-controlled, comparative studies employing the life review method have been published, although unpublished reports have appeared (Carlisle & Molinari, 1980) that lend support to the value of this technique in fostering social interaction, self-esteem, and awareness of maladaptive behavior patterns.

CHAPTER IX

BEHAVIORAL THERAPY
APPROACHES

Several studies have noted the lack of research specifically focusing on the application of behavior therapy techniques with the elderly (Barnes, Sack & Shore, 1973; Cautela, 1966, 1969; Gottesman et al., 1973; Hoyer, Mishara & Riedel, 1975; Knight, 1979; Richards & Thorpe, 1978). Perhaps one of the major reasons for this is the tendency of most behaviorally oriented therapies to ignore age per se as a variable related to outcome of therapy (Gendlin & Rychlak, 1970; Krasner, 1971). As Richards & Thorpe (1978) observed, there has been little preoccupation with the impact of chronological age or "psychosocial stages" upon treatment outcome. This philosophy was also promulgated by Corby (1975) who maintained that techniques and methods emphasizing behavior therapy were tailored to fit specific problems rather than specific populations.

Nevertheless, Gottesman et al. (1973) concluded that age per se does not limit the potential effectiveness of such techniques as positive reinforcement, desensitization, aversive counterconditioning, and modelling. This view has been echoed by other authors with varying orientations to psychotherapy (Ingebretson, 1977; Kastenbaum, 1978). Gottesman et al. (1973) praised behaviorally oriented research that has attempted to empirically determine the variables responsible for influencing therapy outcome. Although they lamented the failure to consider age as a potentially potent variable in this research, Gottesman et al. (1973) observed that the elderly in general should not explicitly be excluded as appropriate candidates for behavioral therapy.

Richards & Thorpe (1978) concluded a review of the current status of behavioral therapy methods with the elderly with several pertinent observations. They first noted that the problems of late life per se have generated no specific treatment techniques, and that there are few controlled studies of behavior therapy conducted with elderly groups. In addition, what studies are available have been relatively unsophisticated and have for the most part ignored more recent theoretical developments and treatments such as biofeedback, cognitive-behavioral techniques, and multi-modal therapy. While it was observed that where comparative data does exist behavior therapy techniques that have been successful with younger populations seem effective with the elderly, Richards & Thorpe (1978) contended that behavioral treatment methods may require modifications for use with the elderly, particularly chronic, institutionalized patients. These authors cited a need for research that will more precisely specify what kinds of modifications should be made in particular techniques when applied to particular behavioral problems.

The lack of sufficient research focusing on behavioral treatment of depression in the elderly seems more regrettable in light of the many potential advantages this orientation offers. Brink (1979) and Richards & Thorpe (1978) have enumerated several characteristics of an environmentally oriented, problem-solving approach which render it particularly well-suited for the elderly. For example, the behavioral emphasis on therapist activity, de-emphasis on the role of insight, and briefer interventions aimed at specific problems may be preferable when working with older individuals who tend to be less active and less responsive to in-depth efforts aimed at a total restructuring of the personality. In addition, behavioral techniques facilitate the packaging of treatment into small, sequential steps, which an older person may more readily assimilate and carry out. As Gendlin & Rychlak (1970) noted, behavioral therapy tends to be less focused on elaborate hypothetical constructs and more concerned with observable behavior that would be amenable to numerous types of intervention.

Thus, rather than focusing attention exclusively on why an individual may be depressed, behavioral therapy techniques attempt to train the client to engage in behaviors that have less aversive and more rewarding consequences. Unlike traditional psychotherapy, which tends to focus upon the perception and labelling of feelings to promote awareness and understanding, behavioral interventions seek to train the individual to find better means of coping with and eliminating negative emotions and self-statements (Brink, 1979). Knight (1979) observed that the behavioral perspective unites treatment with a process of theory development and provides an alternative to viewing problems of the elderly as biological and irreversible.

In their review of behavioral approaches to treatment of the elderly, Cautela & Mansfield (1977) agreed with this assessment. They argued that behavioral methods were especially appropriate with older people who exhibit greater incidence of organic problems. Unlike traditional therapies, these techniques are more flexible because they do not place excessive reliance upon formal diagnosis as a barometer of treatment outcome. Cautela & Mansfield (1977) and Riedel (1974) noted that anxiety and depressive states, resulting from the cumulative impact of psychosocial stressors and manifested by feelings of loss of control over one's environment, are particularly notable in the elderly and should be amenable to behavorial interventions involving such techniques as desensitization, relaxation training and cognitive, self-control manipulations.

The behavioral perspective has generated several prominent etiological and treatment models of depression (Beck, 1967; Beck, Rush, Shaw & Emery, 1979; Lewinsohn, 1974, 1975; Seligman, 1976, 1978). These have been extensively documented elsewhere (Blaney, 1977); however, for the most part, their clinical application has not involved the elderly. Although it should be possible to extend these approaches to the elderly with minimal modification and similar positive outcomes, the fact remains that such efforts have generally not been undertaken. Although several authors (Gardner & Oei, 1981; Shaw, 1977) have recently addressed the relative efficiency of the behavioral and cognitive models in the treatment of depression, the efficacy of these treatments with the elderly remains an open question.

According to Falloon (1975), the available literature concerning the behavioral treatment of depression in the elderly has largely consisted of several case reports involving use of operant methods with institutionalized patients. Another area of promise has been the use of cognitive-behavioral methods in the remediation of grief or bereavement reactions in elderly outpatients (Gauthier & Marshall, 1977). Knight (1979) cited a case report presented by Flannery (1974) as the only instance of the successful treatment of depression using behavioral techniques in an elderly outpatient. In this study, a multifaceted approach involving contracting was used to treat a seventy-seven-year-old man who exhibited physical and social problems related to grief. Treatment consisted of making therapeutic contacts contingent upon the client following a five-step contract containing means for reducing dependence on medication and increasing the level of appropriate social interactions. Social reinforcers were used to increase positive self-statements and to extinguish socially aversive remarks. The therapist also used prompting, shaping and cognitive restructuring methods in directing discussions of grief-related topics during which the client eventually became able to discuss the death of a close relative. Compliance with the contract was monitored by the client's sister, physician, and pharmacist with the client's consent. Successful treatment outcome was indicated by a reflection in medications used and improvement in observational and self-report measures of depression. The author did not discuss the potential confound between the treatment procedures and dependent measures created by engaging medical personnel in monitoring of patient medication usage, however.

Recently, Gauthier & Marshall (1977) provided a cognitive behavioral analysis of prolonged grief reactions in the elderly. They suggested that excessive withdrawal and depression observed in some bereaved elderly persons could be maintained both by social reinforcement of grief behavior and through a process in which the individual is carefully protected from all reminders of the deceased. In a case study of four elderly persons, Gauthier & Marshall (1977) reported noticeable alleviation of chronic grief with as little as six treatment sessions using a variety of cognitive-behavioral methods. The ages of these clients were not specified. Treatment consisted of teaching relatives and friends the use of appropriate, contingent social reinforcement in order to restructure their responses to the clients' grieving behavior. The clients were also directly exposed to images to help extinguish depressive affects associated with memory, thoughts and feelings concerning their lost loved ones. Although failure to include appropriate control groups significantly weakened the conclusions drawn, this case study does suggest that restructuring techniques can be used to modify depressions in the elderly.

One commendable attempt to shed further light on the application and extension of existing behavioral and cognitive therapy modalities to depressed older persons was recently provided by Hussian & Lawrence (1981). This well-controlled outcome study employed a randomized within-subjects crossover design to compare the relative effectiveness of a social reinforcement, activity-based intervention with a cognitively oriented, structured, problem-solving training approach. Thirty-six depressed residents of a nursing home participated in the study and were randomly assigned to either a social reinforcement (SR), problem-solving (PS), or waiting-list control (WLC) group. Each subject received a total of five 30-minute treatment sessions per week for two weeks. At the end of the initial treatment week however, the 12 subjects in each group were randomly reassigned to a second week of either one or the other therapy conditions. This permitted comparisons among subjects on the basis of their having been exposed to either two consecutive weeks of one treatment alone, or one week each of both methods. This design also contrasted groups differing in the sequence in which both therapy conditions were presented, thus controlling for order and expectancy effects.

Results indicated that following the initial week, both types of therapy (SR & PS) significantly reduced levels of depression and improved hospital adjustment as measured by various self-report and objective rating scales when compared to waiting list controls. However, the most important finding of this study was that, after the second week of treatment only those conditions that had included problem-solving training showed significant reductions in depression compared to controls. Hussian & Lawrence (1981) provided follow-up data, which supported their contention that inclusion of some form of cognitive problem-solving training promoted maintenance of treatment gains and that increased social reinforcement alone was not instrumental in the long-term reduction of depression. It was also noted that these data did not support Lewinsohn's (1974) behavioral concept of depression as the result of low rates of response-contingent positive reinforcement due to reduced activity levels.

Although this research seemed to herald the beginning of efforts to elucidate the differential effectiveness of behavioral approaches to treatment of depression in the institutionalized elderly, additional replication is required in light of several design limitations discussed by the authors. These include the lack of multiple measures of depression, validity problems arising from the initial assessment and diagnostic screening of subjects, failure to assess and control for the differential reinforcement values of various activities engaged in by subjects, and failure to adequately control for the qualitative differences between groups in level of contact and nature of experience with the therapist. Finally, in light of recent suggestions concerning possible biases inherent in conducting research with an institutionalized population (Mintz, Steuer & Jarvik, 1981), it would seem advisable to promote external validity and generalization by using noninstitutionalized, outpatient, depressed elderly population samples in future replications.

In a pilot case study of two elderly hospitalized depressed patients, Falloon (1975) reported favorable outcomes using a multimodal, behaviorally oriented treatment package. In this study, a combination of operant reinforcement techniques, in vivo desensitization and social-skills training was used to effect changes in motor and verbal output, depressive verbalizations, and the expression of anxiety and somatic complaints. Both patients discontinued antidepressant medication and were given physicals upon admission to the hospital. During assessment, interactions and behavior with hospital staff, other patients, and relatives were monitored, and patients were then rated using the Hamilton Rating Scale for Depression (Hamilton, 1960). Treatment procedures were then instituted for a period of twenty days, whereupon contingencies were returned to baseline conditions of reassurance and support for ten days. In the behavioral treatment phase, both patients showed consistent improvement in all verbal, motoric, physical and cognitive domains as reflected by marked reduction in Hamilton Rating Scale scores. When the treatment program was suspended, one patient showed no further lowering of depressive scores, while the other deteriorated markedly, erasing earlier treatment gains. Both patients were then returned to treatment conditions with subsequent improvement and eventual discharge.

Falloon (1975) acknowledged both the lack of adequate controls and dependent measures and indicated that this approach should be limited to cases of severe depression that have not responded to physical treatment or where physical treatment is contraindicated. Another concern was the failure to provide follow-up data concerning generalization and maintenance of treatment gains. Nevertheless, preliminary results obtained with this study suggest that treatment based upon Lewinsohn's (1974, 1975) and Beck's (1972, 1976) theoretical conceptualizations of depression (loss of response-contingent positive reinforcement and negative cognitive evaluation and appraisal of the external environment) are useful when applied to treatment of depression in the elderly that is severe enough to require hospitalization.

Although it seems amply clear that behavioral and cognitive behavioral methods offer a viable approach to the understanding and treatment of depression in the elderly, to date their promise remains largely untested empirically. The little literature available does not reflect the recent advances and current sophistication of behavioral therapy with younger populations and what is available is frought with methodological problems which preclude conclusive interpretation of treatment outcome. One hopes that future research will address this problem by manipulating more stringent designs with adequate control groups and more refined subject selection.

CHAPTER X

GROUP THERAPY APPROACHES

Although reports detailing the use of group therapy methods with geriatric populations began to emerge during the 1950's (Linden, 1953; Pappas, Page & Baker, 1958; Rechtschaffen, 1954; Silver, 1950; Smith, 1951; Wolff, 1956, 1957), it is only relatively recently that such methods have gained recognition as a potentially valuable means of helping the elderly cope with depression (Altholz, 1978). Thus, it is hardly surprising that very little controlled research exists that attempts to establish the usefulness of this modality as applied to the treatment of depression among elderly persons.

In addition, much of the available research has focused upon institutionalized populations (Burnside, 1970; Levy, Derogatis, Gallagher & Gatz, 1980), making it difficult to assess the appropriateness of group interventions for the vast majority of older persons who reside within the community. Although a few articles and some research detailing structured group treatment for the non-institutionalized elderly exist (Lago & Hoffman, 1978; Lewis & Butler, 1974; Petty, Moeller & Campbell, 1976; Waters, Fink & White, 1976) the relative efficacy of these methods has not been directly assessed.

Furthermore, Storandt (1978) has noted that virtually no research has examined particular patient characteristics associated with successful results or compared outcome in group therapy as a function of age. Storandt (1978) also noted that certain modifications of technique might be required in geriatric group therapy because practical, environmentally based issues and problems of daily living may take precedence over interpersonal issues and group dynamics. These views were subsequently reinforced in a discussion of the purpose, function and effects of geriatric group therapy by O'Brien, Johnson & Miller (1979). Nevertheless, numerous authors have supported the idea that, at least on an intuitive basis, group therapy is particularly well-suited for the elderly (Burnside, 1978; Capuzzi & Gross, 1980; Ebersole, 1978; Butler & Lewis, 1977; Levy et al., 1980; Mardoyan & Weis, 1981). Before turning to an evaluation of the literature on the effects of group therapy on depression in the elderly, however, it seems advisable to briefly discuss some of the potential advantages of using group procedures with geriatric clients, bearing in mind the fact that virtually no process or outcome research is currently available to support clinically derived observations.

Karpf (1980) viewed group therapy as an extremely useful treatment approach, particularly within the milieu of the institution. He contended that group treatment afforded the elderly the opportunity to maintain appropriate levels of social activity and achieve adequate reality testing through personal interaction and feedback. In a similar view, Verwoerdt (1976) argued that groups constitute perhaps the best approach to providing therapy for elderly individuals because they enhance a sense of belonging and provide a supportive context in which expression of emotion and feedback concerning mutual problems are encouraged. This conclusion was supported by Lowenthal & Haven (1968) who suggested that the opportunity to share personal feelings is especially beneficial to the elderly who have often lost many social and interpersonal roles, supports and outlets. Mardoyan & Weis (1981) recently outlined the advantages of geriatric group therapy in terms of diminishing several factors that inhibit effective therapeutic progress (i.e., unresolved therapist attitudes towards death and aging, age bias, countertransference), factors which may be particularly evident in conventional, one-to-one therapy.

Wolff (1957) discussed several advantages of group therapy, including the reduction of tendencies towards withdrawal among institutionalized patients, increased socialization, and development of new friendships. He noted that group intervention did not seem to be nearly as anxiety-provoking to geriatric patients as a private office visit, and that group process had a stabilizing effect upon symptoms of excessive dependency, delusions, and paranoia among elderly participants through a type of control-by-consensus. In addition, the proximity of many individuals capable of providing mutual support was felt to promote increased self-confidence and self-esteem.

Capuzzi & Gross (1980) noted that the focus of group therapy depended upon the nature and composition of the particular groups and that different groups often have different problems each requiring a different focus. Despite this, Brink (1979) contended that certain goals transcend most differences among groups and are applicable with virtually all geriatric psychotherapy groups. Several authors (Brink, 1979; Burnside, 1978; Mardoyan & Weis, 1981; Ohlsen, 1977) have recently noted the value of group interactions in facilitating cohesiveness, stimulating sociability, and assisting the life review process as elderly patients are exposed to the life experiences of their cohorts. In addition, Brink (1979) recommended that group work with the elderly be reality-based, focused on specific goals related to current life situations, and attuned to the strengths as well as the limitations of group members. Group therapy should function tò motivate and assist the elderly in how to best use current resources in coping with immediate problems. In structured group interventions that use techniques based upon an educational social learning model (i.e., behavioral rehearsal, role play, guided participation), the importance of providing both positive reinforcement (for evidence of successful coping) and continued support (despite ineffective coping) has also been emphasized (Lago & Hoffman, 1978). Brink (1979) has suggested that the general trend towards structured, pragmatic, group interventions with both a reality orientation and life review focus may serve to enhance the individual's ability to define and set realistic goals while providing continuing reminders of successful coping behaviors exhibited during previous transition phases and life crises.

Silver (1950) was apparently one of the first to attempt group psychotherapy with institutionalized geriatric patients. Seventeen female residents, seventy to eighty years of age, were seen twice weekly over a period of several months. Most had been diagnosed as having senile psychosis, and only one group member was considered overtly depressed. Group process revolved, for the most part, on discussions of patients' desires to go home, but other problems, themes and issues included physical complaints, the "good old days," insecurity due to loneliness and socioeconomic factors, wishful fantasies, and rejection by their families. Improvement was observed in general ward behavior, cleanliness, staff morale, and in reduced overall confusion, although the uncontrolled design of this case report does not permit the attribution of successful outcome to the particular treatment methods used, and one cannot ascertain the particular effectiveness, if any, of any of the various components of the group process. Furthermore, there is no way to establish whether improvement in staff morale was a cause, an effect, or was totally unrelated to the improvement in patient behaviors. Finally, no effort was made to discuss individual responsiveness of patients with differing initial diagnoses, so that improvement of affective status or mood was not specifically addressed.

Linden (1953) published results of a two-year study involving group therapy with 51 female, institutionalized senile patients, and reported that 40 percent of this group met criteria for discharge from the hospital after an average of 54 hours of therapy. A control group of 279 other patients had only a 10 percent discharge rate during a similar period. In the intitial phase of the group, free associations plus uninhibited discussions, and mutual interpretations were promoted. This was gradually supplanted by a rotating method of calling on members for both speaking and biographical questioning. As the group progressed further, group members were encouraged to prepare and present educational talks on topics of group interest. Linden (1953) reported that the prevailing atmosphere of pessimism, inactivity, stagnation and futility began gradually to erode among group members and that mutual support and protectiveness developed as cohesiveness solidified. One major problem with this study, however, was the failure to provide data to indicate that the control and experimental groups used were functionally equivalent; without proper matching of the groups prior to initiation of treatment, outcome cannot be unambiguously interpreted. Another problem was that, although criteria specified for inclusion in the group included the expression of at least a "minimal range of affects," the study did not specifically address changes in mood as a function of treatment. Although no systematic approach was used in therapy, Linden concluded that, given an atmosphere of acceptance, interest, and creative participation, regression is halted as the desire for social stimulation and relationships increases.

Benaim (1957) reported some success using a non-directive, passive therapist style in a group established within a hospital geriatric unit. The group usually consisted of between seven and ten males who met once a week for ninety minutes. In all, 18 patients were treated during a five-month period. The average age was sixty-eight years. Diagnoses varied, but included some patients with major affective disorders (e.g., manic depression). This uncontrolled case report concluded that group sessions, although often stormy, increased sociability and contentment for participants through the gradual development of mutual support and an atmosphere that fostered critical evaluations of members' progress. Again, however, change in affective state was not specifically addressed as a function of participation in the group. Generally speaking, other efforts at group therapy with mostly institutionalized patients (Dubey, 1968; Gralewicz, 1968; Oberleder, 1970; Oradei & Waite, 1974) have followed a similar pattern. While reporting encouraging results in improved social behavior, increased discharge rates, and greater activation and morale, these studies have not typically examined outcome in terms of *depression*.

Nevertheless, some reports do suggest that group therapy can be an effective means of alleviating depressed mood states in elderly persons. Liederman & Liederman (1967) described an outpatient therapy group consisting of 11 individuals aged sixty-two to eighty-six who were referred for deficiency in coping skills. These patients were initially quite reluctant to pursue psychological treatment, and had made repeated contacts with physicians. Eventually, however, a great deal of investment and cohesion developed as the group process was directed towards supporting members through their recurring depressive episodes. The group focused on the crises engendered by disabilities and fears of death and dying. Depression was reduced as coping skills improved and isolation and inactivity lessened. The authors, however, did not provide objective means of assessing the observed changes in depression, and again the lack of appropriate control groups precluded definitive conclusions about the effectiveness of the group treatment.

In another uncontrolled case report, Levine and Schild (1969) recruited a homogeneous group of 12 depressed geriatric outpatients and reported that group therapy resulted in improvements in depressed mood which were linked to the dilution and diffusion of dependency demands. This result was achieved by exposing the universality of depressive feelings among group members. The authors maintained that participation in the group led to increased expressions of empathy and acceptance, and reduced feelings of alienation and rejection. Again, however, no objective data were provided to substantiate findings based on group process.

More recently, an ongoing program of group psychotherapy for elderly outpatients was presented by Deutsch & Kramer (1977). Over a two-year period, approximately ninety referrals to the group were made, mostly due to depression and/or psychosomatic complaints resulting from combinations of physical, mental or social losses. Five time-limited brief therapy groups were established. Each group had a maximum of 12 members who met for 90 minutes once a week for 12 consecutive weeks. Members could request continued participation in subsequent 12-week sessions. The groups had three basic objectives: to emphasize that the aging process is a normal part of the life cycle, to generate positive attitudes and model new behaviors that would increase self-worth, and to help members become involved in meaningful activities regardless of level of physical incapacitation. Sessions generally focused on physical, economic and social losses resulting in grief and/or depression. The authors noted that feelings of uselessness and worthlessness were the common denominator among older persons in crisis. They reported several successful cases in detail and concluded that remarkable improvements in coping skills were attained by members who made a strong commitment to therapy. Deutsch & Kramer (1977) recommended group treatment as a resource for community-based elderly persons on the basis of subjective clinical impression of improvement in coping skills and reductions in depression and withdrawal in social settings. Follow-up data on individual patients in the form of participation in subsequent volunteer activities, part-time jobs, or renewed contacts with family and friends was cited as further evidence of improvement, and provided additional support for the effectiveness of the group experience. Nevertheless, the lack of relevant controls did not permit unequivocal interpretations regarding the relationship between therapy gains and improvement in social functioning or other indices used to gauge level of interpersonal functioning and activation.

Another look at the effect of group therapy on depression was provided by Lazarus (1976), who described a comprehensive and detailed long-term program of group psychotherapy employed at a private inpatient facility. The group program, involving nearly all geriatric patients aged sixty and over, was initiated in 1968 when it became apparent that group programs were employed successfully with young adults and adolescents, while most elderly patients were depressed, isolated, and uninvolved in the hospital milieu program. Lazarus noted that prior to establishment of the therapy program, elderly patients reacted to hospitalization by becoming either extremely withdrawn and resigned or excessively dependent and demanding. Staff reacted to these demands either by gratifying patients' requests (unintentionally fostering increased dependency) or by reacting with frustration and anger (increasing mutual guilt and anxiety). Repetition of this uneasy cycle of accomodation followed by anger and avoidance led to decreased staff concern for the elderly and fostered increased regression, withdrawal, and avoidance in the patients. Group therapy was then instituted to enhance resocialization and eliminate regressed behavior. Butler's (1960) theory that elderly patients could benefit from interpretation, confrontation and support was also tested.

Group therapy was made available for all patients aged sixty and over. Groups were usually comprised of between four and twelve individuals. Average length of hospital stay for group members was 34 days. The average age was seventy-four and ranged from sixty-nine to eighty-nine. Based on his total statistical analysis, Lazarus (1976) reported that in an average group of nine patients, seven were typically hospitalized because of severe depression, and that one-third of the patients received primarily electroshock therapy, with the remainder receiving psychotherapy. Treatment was provided by a team consisting of a psychiatric resident, occupational therapist, social worker and nurse. Patients were evaluated for group candidacy by interviews upon admission, and were recommended by the treatment team after staffing and supervision. Only patients manifesting uncontrollable aggression were excluded. Patients invited to participate attended group twice weekly for 30 minutes. A dinner with wine was held for group members once weekly to foster cohesion and identity, and was also used to give those patients uncertain about joining the group the chance to become better acquainted.

Lazarus (1976) noted that one of the major presenting symptoms was depression, usually secondary to the loss of a loved object and/or awareness of a deterioration of ego-functioning. Group members typically exhibited defenses such as withdrawal from interpersonal relationships and preoccupation with somatic complaints. Passive defense mechanisms were employed as a means of dealing with anxiety and fears of death. Members' anger towards their children because of actual or perceived rejection was often displaced onto other group members. Ambivalent feelings toward deceased spouses often were expressed by self-punishment and blame. These dynamics underscored the typical patient's prevailing attitude of hopelessness, despair, isolation and fears for the future.

The strategies and goals of the group intervention outlined by Lazarus (1976) took several forms. Therapists employed careful listening, empathy, and positive feedback to communicate acceptance and concern. Suggestions were given to group members about ways of effecting changes within their milieu. Responses to patients' dependency demands were initially made and then faded out in the attempt to support the individual's own resourcefulness and abilities in problem solving. Fears and anxieties were addressed and diminished through reassurances and educational explanations provided by other patients and therapists. Perhaps most important, members were encouraged to reminisce about past crises and accomplishments. Lazarus (1976) contended that this upsurge of long buried memories seemed to alleviate depression stemming from current problems, and promote pride in past achievements while instilling renewed confidence and hope for the future. Group cohesion and support also served to alleviate the depressive tone surrounding explanations of sentiments regarding death, dying, and loss of loved ones. Further, therapists employed empathic questioning and confrontation in response to patients' expressions of guilt and self-blame for past mistakes and "crimes."

Lazarus (1976) discussed problems encountered in implementing group therapy attributable to both patients and therapists. It was noted that for many elderly patients, hospitalization often follows long periods of isolation, depression, withdrawal and despair, and symbolically represents a turning point that raises the spectre of ultimate decline leading to death. The elderly patient craves group contact while also avoiding it for fear of further rejection or abandonment. Group process and cohesiveness was often interrupted due to turnover among members; it resulted in frequent discussions centered on themes of loss and separation. Another potential problem was described in terms of transference reactions on the part of group members—reactions that often precipitated rivalries among them for the attention of the therapists. These were usually not interpreted but were utilized instead to help patients form improved relationships with each other. Therapists often had to handle expressions of anger and disappointment as patients reacted to the failure of their exaggerated transference expectations.

In evaluating therapists' contributions to the group process, Lazarus (1976) observed an initial tendency on their part to be too hasty in gratifying demands and to compete among themselves for patients' acceptance. He noted that too much support and reassurance fostered continued regressive behavior, and that giving in to unrealistic demands merely exacerbated the patients' sense of decline and dependency, which further eroded self-esteem. Lazarus (1976) stressed that patients generally responded more favorably to clarification, confrontation and interpretation, and some were able to achieve insight into how present interpersonal conflicts were extensions of past relationships with significant others. The therapeutic approach used varied for each individual group member depending upon the therapist's appraisal of patient dynamics and level of autonomous functioning. Therefore, supportive techniques such as reassurance and guidance were employed where patients were judged unable to benefit significantly from more insight-oriented techniques.

The major shortcoming of Lazarus' (1976) program was the lack of objective, strict, clinical criteria and control groups to determine relative effectiveness of the therapy program. Furthermore, there were no dependent measures of improvement in depression which supposedly was a major objective and reported outcome of treatment. Lazarus (1976) argued that the principle value of the group program was the atmosphere of acceptance and trust that enabled patients to increase their self-esteem and resulted in renewed social relationships and improved ego-functioning. The resocialization aspects of the group process encouraged recovery and utilization of former social abilities and skills and helped dispel feelings of isolation and despair. Thus, despite similarities between earlier group therapy programs with hospitalized geriatric patients demonstrating improvement in both affect and social behaviors, Lazarus' research (1976) regrettably failed to apply rigorous experimental controls and procedures for quantifying overt changes in affective state, leaving the question of the precise relationship between group therapy and outcome of depression unanswered.

Recently, several comparative outcome studies examining the efficacy of different group therapy approaches have included changes in depression or related psychological variables as outcome measures (Gallagher, 1979; Ingersoll & Silverman, 1978). In Gallagher's (1979) controlled research, behavioral group therapy was compared with a non-directive group therapy. It was found that the elderly responded about equally well to both approaches. Results showed that although the behavioral therapy group yielded greater improvement in verbal interaction in group sessions, improvements in self-report measures of depression or interpersonal behavior showed no significant differences as a function of type of treatment received. These findings suggest perhaps that many non-specific effects such as subject expectancies and experimental demand characteristics could have operated to influence outcome. This study suggests that the process of group interaction may be more important than the specific focus, methods and structure of the group. Carefully devised placebo, nontreatment, and activity control groups are essential in order to properly evaluate differential treatment responses to group therapy.

Lack of different treatment effects due to non-specific factors was also observed in the Ingersoll & Silverman (1978) comparative outcome research. In this study, the effects of a "there and then" reminiscence-oriented outpatient group was compared with a "here and now" behaviorally oriented group. The "here and now" approach was based on the behavioral learning theory model which regards excessive focusing on the past or future as maladaptive. The therapy approach stemming from this model was geared to offer specific, pragmatic help for specific problems rather than attempting to uncover past conflicts. This reflected a behavioral focus on present-oriented, concrete problem solving. The basic rationale of the "here and now" method presumed that decreasing anxiety would improve self-esteem and reduce somatic complaints. The "there and then" group in this study used an insight-oriented approach that utilized reminiscing.

Several theorists (Butler, 1970; Kramer, Kramer & Dunlop, 1966; Pincus, 1970) have hypothesized that reminiscing is an adaptive process that increases self-esteem, facilitates a sense of identity, promotes coping with personal losses and decreases depression.

Subjects for the experiment were recruited through various media advertisements. Adults over sixty experiencing tension, depression, memory lapses or insomnia were encouraged to participate. Clients were randomly assigned to treatment groups. Both groups in the study were quite similar in composition, and no matching along subject variables was undertaken. According to Ingersoll & Silverman (1978) every subject was experiencing anxiety or depression due to age-related losses. Dependent measures were based on pre- and post-tests on self-report questionnaires tapping self-esteem, anxiety and somatic complaints. Interestingly, although depression was a primary intervention target, the authors apparently did not use measures specifically designed to tap changes in mood. Other outcome information was gathered through clinical progress notes from each session, and a debriefing telephone interview one week following termination. Apparently depression was only indirectly assessed through a self-esteem score and through subjective impressions based on interview and progress-note data.

Each group met once a week for a total of eight two-hour sessions. The major emphasis in the "here and now" behavioral group was on developing awareness of body tension and training in progressive muscle relaxation. Behavioral techniques such as modelling, reinforcement and role playing were used to help clients deal with memory loss, boredom and depression. Depression was only focused on specifically during the sixth or seventh sessions. Subjects were asked to develop and share a list of high-frequency, highly rewarding activities to self-monitor during the ensuing week. The hope was that this would result in an increased frequency of such activities.

The major emphasis in the insight-oriented group was on reminiscing and the life review process. Clients were encouraged to keep journals and construct genograms that trace family origins. Sessions revolved around sharing earliest memories and the recognition of family and personal behavior patterns. Regrets over past mistakes were paired with remembrances of past achievements and accomplishments. Depression was addressed primarily through discussion of significant losses during the construction of the genogram.

Results based on change scores indicated that while the insight "there and then" group showed greater overall improvements at the conclusion of the study, only one measured difference between groups (i.e., somatic complaints) reached statistical significance. The authors suggested that the time required by elderly persons to learn the behavioral techniques used in the "here and now" group may have exceeded the time frame allotted for the experiment. Another design problem was the lack of suitable no-treatment activity and waiting list control groups, which made it difficult to evaluate the potential effects of extraneous variables and nonspecific symptoms changes (i.e., spontaneous recovery, placebo effects, experimental demand characteristics) on the results. Ingersoll & Silverman (1978) concluded that the lack of significant differential improvement between groups suggests that the particular therapy method employed may be irrelevent, as long as the elderly are given the opportunity to interact with peers in a supportive context. Thus, it is not possible to determine at present whether lack of definitive results reflects weak method and flawed design or whether treatments were actually not equally effective. The uncontrolled nature of this study does not preclude making a cognitive behavioral interpretation for outcomes and behavioral changes observed in the insight treatment group. The insight group may have actually fostered increased positive self-evaluation and self-reinforcement as a by-product of having clients engage in pleasureable, reinforcing activities. This in turn may have altered levels of anxiety and improved self-esteem by promoting independence and dispelling the sense of helplessness that prevailed before treatment. Ultimately there may be no way to eliminate the interpretation that behavioral mechanisms were actually responsible for producing the changes observed in the insight-oriented group.

Partial support for this possibility has been provided by a recent study with several ambitious objectives (Harris & Bodden, 1978). This research was designed to assess the effectiveness of a structured activation and socialization group intervention in improving psychological adjustment and emotional well-being in a group of withdrawn, community-residing older persons defined as having largely disengaged from society. In addition, this study compared and tested the tenets of activity and disengagement theories, the two main differing viewpoints concerning the necessary and sufficient conditions for successful adaptation to late life. They found that disengaged elderly subjects exposed to the activity-group intervention demonstrated significant improvement when compared with no-treatment controls on most indices of psychological functioning. Furthermore, these individuals approached and maintained the level of functioning exhibited by a pre-selected, baseline reference control group comprised of elderly persons with a high current level of activity, engagement and community involvement. These results suggest that the reinforcing events and activities provided within any group context (such as the insight group of the Ingersoll & Silverman 1978 study) may be the active ingredients responsible for fostering increased adaptation and enhanced emotional stability in the elderly.

Perhaps the most glaring deficiency of the Ingersoll & Silverman (1978) research was the lack of any direct assessment of depression—despite an obvious intention to focus on changes in affective status. Although self-esteem was measured and found to increase in subjects regardless of group assignment, the authors never indicated the extent, if any, to which this measure was intended to correlate with depression, and they did not provide an objective demonstration of changes in depressed mood. It was noted that more elaborately controlled research would be required to identify the specific elements in group therapy responsible for behavior change. Levy et al. (1980) argued that this effort was justified, but cautioned that outcome measures would require further refinement in order to distinguish specific treatment effects from non-specific change.

Despite these shortcomings, one noteworthy aspect of the Ingersoll & Silverman (1978) study was its intentional incorporation of the life-review approach and reminiscence in a group context as a means of overcoming depression. The basic features of the life review have already been described above as a potentially valuable method of individual therapy with the elderly. Advocates of this approach have suggested that it may be quite effectively applied in group therapy settings, and they have outlined several of its therapeutic advantages (Butler & Lewis, 1977; Capuzzi & Gross,

1980; Ebersole, 1978; Lewis & Butler, 1974). Reminiscing in a group situation can facilitate a positive cohort effect enabling members to share both positive and negative aspects of aging. Through this process group members can be helped to achieve a revitalized sense of personal worth and self respect, as stereotypes that equate advanced age with disintegration and disgrace are dispelled. The mutual exchange of early life memories and accomplishments builds rapport and unity while promoting increased socialization and communication skills. Re-creation of pleasurable past events and remembrances of prior successes and achievements are potential sources of positive reinforcement. The process can facilitate awareness that the individual is still capable of displaying resourcefulness and employing successful coping strategies to overcome current problems.

In one variation of the life review approach, the value of employing heterogeneous age groups has been advocated as a means of minimizing the sense of age isolation many elderly individuals experience (Butler, 1964; Butler & Lewis, 1977). Whereas groups comprised of only aged persons often tend to focus on illness, death and loneliness, age integrated groups allow for a broader perspective and the examination of concerns related to intergenerational relationships. This exposure to younger generations can promote awareness of both continuity and adaptation in the process of changes in all phases of the life cycle. This approach can enable elderly group members to re-experience the past through the experiences of younger generations, because these different age groups symbolically recapitulate the family's way of dealing with life crises.

Although Lewis & Butler (1974) reported an ongoing

investigation of age-integrated, life-review group therapy dating to 1970, their data consisted almost exclusively of clinical case reports and observations. There was no assessment of individuals using objectively defined, quantifiable indices of behavioral or affective status. Global clinical impressions (rather than specific outcome comparisons) were the only data reported. Thus, with one or two possible exceptions there have been, to date, no detailed, well controlled outcome studies comparing the relative efficacy of life review to other forms of group therapy (Ingersoll & Silverman, 1978; Lazarus, 1976). Furthermore, there has been little basic research conducted to determine which, if any, of the components used in life review group therapy may be actively responsible for treatment effects and which are clinically inert. It should be pointed out, however, that a similar problem besets psychotherapy outcome research regardless of factors such as age of population, type of psychopathology manifested, or theoretical orientation and therapeutic strategy employed (Mintz et al. 1981; Phillips & Bierman, 1981; Rounsaville, Weissman & Prusoff, 1981).

CHAPTER XI

CONCLUSIONS AND RECOMMENDATIONS

We have documented the use of psychotherapy in the treatment of depression in the elderly, and considered various diagnostic issues and phenomenological questions relevant to depression. The salient aspects of these issues are presented below as a model of late-life depression and integrated with an analysis of some problems besetting psychotherapy research in this area.

The studies surveyed here have provided strong evidence that the elderly are disproportionately subject to emotional and physical problems and are often least likely to seek or be provided with appropriate psychological treatment. The fact that depression constitutes the most common emotional problem exhibited by the elderly has sparked ongoing debate as to whether it is an inevitable consequence of aging, or if, indeed, it may represent a positive, adaptive coping response to the normal decline associated with the aging process. These questions are important, for, as demand for geriatric mental health services will be likely to increase dramatically in the future, professionals and paraprofessional service providers alike will need to be aware of the issues and techniques of psychotherapy that have emerged as a result of previous experiences with geriatric populations. One major issue has been the question of whether or not the elderly are amenable to psychotherapy. This book has reviewed the negative stereotypes and prejudicial biases held by society at large, as well as by therapists, and has detailed considerable evidence demonstrating that, under most circumstances, virtually all forms of psychotherapy reportedly have been useful with the elderly in ameliorating depression and other emotional dysfunction.

Several issues related to the problems associated with the diagnosis and treatment of depression in the elderly were subsequently evaluated. The evidence surveyed strongly supported the idea that depression is a complex disorder which is often difficult to classify definitively in any age group and particularly in the elderly. This may be because, as numerous authors have argued, the elderly are a far more heterogeneous population than the young merely by virtue of their having traversed more of the life span (Butler & Lewis, 1977; Fassler & Gaviria, 1978; Kastenbaum, 1978). Contrary to impressions created by negative cultural stereotypes, the elderly are not a homogeneous group.

Indeed, they tend to exhibit increasing diversity as a function of advancing age. Furthermore, as Epstein (1976) noted, a single, primary cause of depression is unlikely to be identifiable in the elderly. The fulmination of depression in this group appears to be an intricate interaction between past experience, current environmental circumstances, level of current adaptation and coping skills, changing physical status and emergent psychological and sociological stressors.

The difficulties inherent in assessing these factors are further compounded by the similarity between many of the symptoms of depression with other forms of psychopathology, physical ailments or chronic brain syndromes, all of which tend to be more prevalent in elderly populations. The need for an exhaustive analysis of all relevant biological, psychological and social conditions contributing to the elderly individual's level of adaptive functioning was repeatedly stressed as an important means of determining whether symptoms of depression actually represent serious pathology or whether depression is merely a realistic, adaptive coping response to sudden and continuing life-cycle changes. Serious deficiencies or breakdowns in any of these areas should be isolated as targets for possible intervention because, if left untreated, they may deepen transient depression, which may be a normal part of the aging process.

Another related question with profound implications for the manner in which late-life depression is viewed and which, in turn, directly influences the conduct of psychotherapy, concerns whether or not depression is phenomenologically similar across the life span. The available evidence overwhelmingly reinforces the impression that there are few, if any, marked qualitative differences that distinguish *early-* from *late-*onset depression. In this review we have suggested that it is more reasonable to view personality organization, and hence the expression of psychopathology, as qualitatively similar across the life span, and that too much emphasis is placed upon chronological age rather than upon the specific problems of individuals, which may or may not be a consequence of age. It has been the contention of numerous authors (Butler & Lewis, 1977; Goldstein, 1979; Kastenbaum, 1978; Neugarten, 1973; Solomon, 1981; Vickers, 1976; Willner, 1978) that personality organization is the pivotal factor in predicting successful adaptation and coping in old age. Such a model suggests that those individuals who typically reacted to stress in early life by becoming depressed are more likely to experience depression as a result of increased adaptational requirements imposed by the aging process.

We favor a synthesis of opposing views, for in reality they are not irreconcilable. There is a qualitative similarity of depression throughout the life span. In addition, the nature of the external and internal conditions thought to precipitate depression may also be similar regardless of Age. Differences emerge because in old age there may be an ever increasing accumulation of these precipitating factors, which may overwhelm the adaptive capacity of the individual. The cumulative influence of multiple losses and stressors in the biological, psychological and sociological domains imparts a quantitative dimension to aging which emphasizes that, while the life experience of the patient may change with the passage of time, the expression of depressive symptoms remains fairly constant. This approach emphasizes that therapy should be based on the nature of the pathology and not primarily upon the age of a patient. Nevertheless, as previously noted, therapy techniques used in treating depression in the elderly may require modifications that incorporate the quantitative changes associated with advanced age and recognize the wide variability in current levels of adaptations.

It was also demonstrated that the adaptive coping skills of the elderly are often severely challenged as former sources of self-esteem and positive reinforcement (such as cognitive functions and physical abilities) gradually undergo the cumulative erosion of normal biological aging. In this context, the themes of loss and disengagement were discussed as socioeconomic concomitants of late-life depression. This review explored the relationship between various forms of loss incurred by the individual and the possible effects these have in producing a sense of helplessness, role-lessness and decreased control over the environment, all of which may lead to depression. While no formal equation for analyzing these relationships presently exists, it is vitally important to assess each individual case to determine the number and nature of losses involved in order to plan suitable intervention strategies and formulate appropriate, realistic therapy goals.

Disengagement was another major sociological factor associated with depression in the elderly. Inconsistencies in theories of disengagement were noted in order to reveal that, although disengagement may characterize the psychological functioning of some elderly depressed individuals, it is not necessarily a prerequisite of successful aging. Before reaching firm conclusions about the role of disengagement in creating or exacerbating depression, the therapist must consider the extent and mutuality of the disengagement between individual and environment, and assess the indivdual's satisfaction with the arrangement.

Personality constructs and cognitive processes are also potentially implicated in late-life depressions. The ideas of geriatric rigidity and personal locus of control were discussed. Although rigidity is often associated with inadequate adaptation, it is uncertain whether rigidity plays a causal role. It was suggested that rigidity may represent a coping strategy employed by the aged as a means of defending against increased social and physiological debilitation. Similarly, the concept of locus of control was shown to be particularly appropriate as a description of processes leading to depression in geriatric populations. Solomon (1981) has echoed previous work by Goldfarb (1974) in noting the relationship between loss of personal control and depression in the elderly. The aging process typically results in a corresponding shift of authority over personal life events and a greater reliance upon external sources for essential needs. This dissipation of personal control fosters increased dependency which may in turn significantly increase the risk of depression for older persons. In this model, therapy must address the personal helplessness, rolelessness and alienation in the elderly depressive by undermining the influence of any existing negative societal and cultural stereotypes and inhibitions that may be serving to reinforce depressive behavior and symptoms.

The major portion of this review detailed the relative effectiveness of different methods of psychotherapy that have been applied to the treatment of geriatric depression. The bulk of this literature suggested that— irrespective of the particular style, orientation, or methodology—psychotherapy invariably was reported to be capable of producing discernible and often significant improvement in alleviating depression in elderly clients. In particular, the merits of short-term, focused, directive and supportive methods were noted. Training in problem-solving skills and other cognitive-behavioral interventions are potentially quite adaptable for use with the elderly and have the added benefit of being empirically based and easily subject to verification and revision through ongoing outcome and process research. Regrettably, such research efforts have as yet been quite sparse. Finally, it should be noted that more traditionally oriented therapies and those employing a "there and then," reminiscent approach have often been as effective as more "here and now," behaviorally oriented methods.

Unfortunately, this sense of an across-the-board optimism may be premature, as perhaps the most consistent pattern to emerge from this review has been the notable lack of systematic, well-controlled outcome research to substantiate these favorable impressions. The status of geriatric psychotherapy research is, at best, in its infancy. In a brief article, Mintz et al. (1981) outlined several important methodological, practical, and ethical considerations for conducting psychotherapy research with depressed elderly patients. Many of these had already been discussed in the context of addressing diagnostic and phenomenological issues related to geriatric depression. They include, in part, the myth or stereotype of the homogeneity of elderly patients, the difficulty in distinguishing between symptoms produced by depression and those caused by the presence of physical disorders, the potential complications of medical treatment and drug interactions which may either mimic or mask signs of depression, and the realization that characteristic changes of the aging process may require modification of therapy stategies of elderly patients. Other previously defined problems in implementation of research have arisen from failure to consider the impact of therapists' experience, age, and attitudes towards the elderly. Another major difficulty hindering psychotherapy research with the elderly is the absence of adequate normative data for the classification of psychopathology in older populations. Many measurements of adult personal and social adjustment are not valid for use with them. For example, scales of stressful life events should be used with caution because their construction biases them in favor of identifying depression in older populations. Several other potential sources of bias in the design and conduct of psychotherapy research with depressed elderly patients include the failure to adequately investigate reasons for treatment dropout, failure to secure adequate follow-up data, and the failure to ensure the representativeness and generalizabilty of patient populations.

Despite these problems, it is increasingly apparent that pessimism regarding the potential responsiveness of the elderly to psychotherapy is rapidly eroding. An emergent optimism is gradually taking hold as the awareness grows that, in many cases, psychotherapy constitutes an acceptable and viable alternative to reliance on pharmacological or other methods of treatment. It is imperative that research be accelerated, not only to evaluate and refine existing psychotherapy methods, but to facilitate the development of more effective strategies that will meet the needs imposed by shifts in cultural attitudes and demographic trends. It is only in this matter that geriatric psychotherapy, currently in its infancy, will blossom to full maturity.

REFERENCES

Abraham, K. The applicability of psychoanalytic treatment to patients at an advanced age. In K. Abraham, *Selected papers of psychoanalysis*. London: Hogarth Press, 1949.

Abraham, K. *Selected papers of Karl Abraham*. New York: Basic Books. 1927.

Akiskal, H. S. The pathogenesis of depressive disorders. In R. A. Depue, ed., *The psychobiology of the depressive disorders: Implications for the effects of stress*. New YOrk: Academic Press, 1978.

Akiskal, H. S., & McKinney, W. T. Overview of recent research in depression: Ten conceptual models. *Archives of General Psychiatry*, 1975, 32, 285-305.

143

Alexander, F. G. the indications for psychoanalytic therapy. *Bulletin of the New York Academy of Medicine*, 1944, *20*, 319-334.

Alexander, F. G., & French, T. M. *Psychoanalytic therapy: Principles and applications.* New York: Ronald Press, 1946.

Altholz, J. Group therapy with elderly patients. In E. Pfeiffer, ed. *Alternatives to institutional care for older Americans: Practice and planning.* Durham, N. C.: Duke University, Center for the Study of Aging and Human Development, 1978.

Arieti, S. A psychotherapeutic approach to severely depressed patients. *American Journal of Psychotherapy*, 1978, *32*, 33-47.

Bandura, A. Self-efficacy: Toward a unifying theory of behavioral change. *Psychological Review*, 1977, *84*, 191-215.

Barnes, E., Sack, A., & Shore, H. Guidelines to treatment approaches: Modalities and methods for use with the aged. *The Gerontologist*, 1973, *13*, 513-527.

Beck, A. T. *Cognitive theory and the emotional disorders.* New York: International Universities Press, 1976.

Beck, A. T. *Depression: Clinical, experimental and theoretical aspects.* New York: Harper & Row, 1967.

Beck, A. T., Rush, A., Shaw, B., & Emergy, G. *Cognitive therapy of depression: A treatment manual.* New York: Guilford, 1979.

Bell, J. Z. Disengagement versus engagement: A need for greater expectations. *Journal of the American Geriatrics Society*, 1978, *26*, 89-95.

Benaim, S. Group psychotherapy within a geriatric unit: An experiment. *International Journal of Social Psychiatry*, 1957, *3*, 123-128.

Bennett, A. E. Psychiatric management of geriatric depressive disorders. *Diseases of the Nervous System*, 1973, *34* 222-225.

Benson, R. The forgotten treatment modality in bipolar illness: Psychotherapy. *Diseases of the Nervous System*, 1975, *36*, 634-638.

Berezin, M. A. Psychodynamic considerations of aging and the aged: An overview. *American Journal of Psychiatry*, 1972, *128*, 1483-1491.

Berezin, M. A., & Cath, S. H. *Geriatric psychiatry*. New York: International Universities Press, 1965.

Bibring, E. The mechanism of depression. In P. Greenacre, ed. *Affective disorders*. New York: International Universities Press, 1953.

Birren, J. E. *The psychology of aging*. Englewood Cliffs, N. J.: Prentice Hall, 1964.

Blaney, P. H. Contemporary theories of depression: Critique and comparison. *Journal of Abnormal Psychology*, 1977, *86*, 203-223.

Blank, M. L. Raising the age barrier to psychotherapy. *Geriatrics*, 1974, *29*, 141-148.

Blau, D., & Berezin, M. A. Neurosis in character disorder. In J. G. Howells, ed. *Modern perspectives in the psychiatry of old age*. London: Churchill Livingstone, 1975.

Blum, J. E., & Tallmer, M. The therapist vis-à-vis the older patient. *Psychotherapy: Research and Practice*, 1977, *14*, 361-366.

Blumenthal, M. D. Measuring depressive symptomatology in general population. *Archives of General Psychiatry*, 1975, *32*, 971.

Bok, M. Some problems in milieu treatment of the chronic older mental patient. *The Gerontologist*, 1971, *11*, 141-147.

Bornstein, P. F., Clayton, P. J., Halikas, J. A., Maurice, W. L., & Robins, E. The depression of widowhood after thirteen months. *British Journal of Psychiatry*, 1973, *122*, 561-566.

Botwinick, J. *Aging and behavior*. New York: Springer, 1973.

Braceland, F. J. Stresses that cause depression in middle life. *Geriatrics*, 1972, *27*, 45-46.

Brink, T. L. Brief psychotherapy: A case report illustrating its potential effectiveness. *Journal of the American Geriatrics Society*, 1977, *25*, 273-276.

Brink, T. L. *Geriatric psychotherapy*. New York: Human Sciences Press, 1979.

Brink, T. L. Geriatric regidity and its psychotherapeutic implications. *Journal of the American Geriatrics Society*, 1978, *26*, 274-277.

Brody, E. M., Kleban, M. H., Lawton, M. P., & Silverman, H. A. Excess disabilities of mentally impaired aged: Impact of individualized treatment. *Gerontologist*, 1971, *2*, 124-133.

Burnside, I. M. Group work with the aged: Selected literature. *Gerontologist*, 1970, *10*, 241-246.

Burnside, I. M. Longterm group work with hospitalized aged. *Gerontologist*, 1971m *11*, 213-218.

Burnside, I. M., ed. *Working with the elderly: Group process and techniques*. North Scituate, Mass.: Duxbury Press, 1978.

Busse, E. W. Hypchondriasis in the elderly. *Journal of the American Geriatrics Society*, 1976, *24*, 145-149.

Busse, E. W. Research on aging: Some methods of findings. In M. A. Berezin & S. H. Cath, eds. *Geriatric psychiatry: Grief, loss and emotional disorders in the aging process*. New York: International Universities Press, 1965.

Busse, E. W. Treatment of the non-hospitalized, emotionally disturbed elderly person. *Geriatrics*, 1971, *11*, 175-179.

Busse, E. W., Barnes, R. H., Silverman, A. J., Thaler, M., & Frost, L. L. Studies of the process of aging. X: The strength and weakness of psychic functioning in the aged. *American Journal of Psychiatry*, 1955, *111*, 896-903.

Busse, E. W., & Pfeiffer, E. Functional psychiatric disorders in old age. In E. W. Busse & E. Pfeiffer, eds., *Behavior and adaptation in late life*. Boston: Little, Brown & Co., 1977.

Busse, E. W., & Pfeiffer, E. *Mental illness in later life*. Washington, D. C.: American Psychiatric Association, 1973.

Butler, R. Intensive psychotherapy for the hospitalized aged. *Geriatrics*, 1960, *15*, 644-653.

Butler, R. Life review. In R. J. Kastenbaum, ed., *New thoughts on old age*. New York: Springer, 1964.

Butler, R. Successful aging and the role of the life review. *American Geriatrics Society*, 1970, *12*, 529-532.

Butler, R. Psychiatry and the elderly: An overview. *American Journal of Psychiatry*, 1975, *132*, 893-900.

Butler, R., & Lewis, M. *Aging and mental health*. St. Louis: Mosby Co., 1973.

Butler, R., & Lewis, M. *Aging and mental health*. St. Louis: Mosby Co., 1977.

Cabeen, C. W., & Coleman, J. C. The selection of sex-offender patients for group psychotherapy. *International Journal of Group Psychotherapy*, 1962, *12*, 326-334.

Capuzzi, D., & Gross, D. Group work with the elderly: An overview for counselors. *Personnel and Guidance Journal*, 1980, *59*, 206-211.

Carlisle, A. & Molinari, V. *A life review course for the elderly*. Unpublished manuscript, Texas Research Institute of Mental Sciences, 1980.

Cartwright, D. S. Success in psychotherapy as a function of certain actuarial variables. *Journals of Consulting Psychology*, 1955, *19*, 357-363.

Carver, E. J. Geropsychiatric treatment: Where, why, how. In W. E. Fann & G. L. Maddox, eds., *Drug issues in geropsychiatry*. Baltimore: Williams & Wilkins, 1974.

Cath, S. Psychoanalytic viewpoints on aging: An historical survey. In D. P. Kent, R. Kastenbaum & S. Sherwood, eds., *Research planning and action for the elderly*. New York: Behavioral Publications, 1972.

Cautela, J. R. Behavior therapy and geriatrics. *Journal of Genetic Psychology*, 1966, *108*, 9-17.

Cautela, J. R. A classical conditioning approach to the development and modification of behavior in the aged. *The Gerontologist*, 1969, *9*, 109-113.

Cautela, J. R., & Mansfield, L. A behavioral approach to geriatrics. In W. D. Gentry, ed., *Geropsychology: A model of training and clinical service*. Cambridge: Ballinger, 1977.

Charatan, F. B. Depression in old age. *New York State Journal of Medicine*, 1975, 2505-2509.

Corby, N. Assertion training with aged populations. *The Counselling Psychologist*, 1975, *5*, 69-74.

Covi, L., Lipman, R., Derogatis, L., Smith, V., & Pattison, J. Drugs and group psychotherapy in neurotic depression. *American Journal of Psychiatry*, 1974, *131*, 191-198.

Cox, J. R., Pearson, R., & Brand, H. Lithium in depression. *Gerontology*, 1977, *23*, 219-235.

Cumming, E. Further thoughts on the theory of disengagement. *International Social Science Journal*, 1963, *15*, 337-393.

Cumming, E. New thoughts on the theory of disengagement. In R. Kastenbaum, ed., *New thoughts on old age*. New York: Springer, 1964.

Cumming, E., & Henry, W. E. *Growing old: The process of disengagement*. New York: Basic Books, 1961.

Cumming, J., & Cumming, E. Care in the community. In J. G. Howells, ed., *Modern perspectives in the psychiatry of old age*. Edinburgh: Churchill Livingstone, 1975.

Da Silva, G. The loneliness and death of an old man. *Journal of Geriatric Psychiatry*, 1967, *1*.

Davis, J. M. Overview: maintenance therapy in psychiatry: II. Affective disorders. *The American Journal of Psychiatry*, 1976, *133*, 1-13.

Davis, R. W., & Klopfer, W. G. Issues in psychotherapy with the aged. *Psychotherapy: Theory, Research and Practice*, 1977, *14*, 343-348.

Deutsch, C. B., & Kramer, N. Outpatient group psychotherapy for the elderly: An alternative to institutionalization. *Hospital & Community Psychiatry*, 1977, *28*, 440-442.

Donahue, W. Psychological aspects. In E. V. Cowdry & F. U. Steinberg, eds. *Care of the geriatric patient*, 4th edition. St. Louis: Mosby, 1971.

Dovenmuehle, R. H., Reckless, J. B., Newman, G. Depressive reactions in the elderly. In *Normal againg*. Durham, N. C.: Duke University Press, 1970.

Dubey, E. Intensive treatment of the institutionalized ambulatory geriatric patient. *Geriatrics*, 1968, *23*, 170-177.

Ebersole, P. P. Establishing reminiscing groups. In I.

M. Burnside, ed., *Working with the elderly: Group process and techniques*. North Scituate Mass.: Duxbury Press, 1978.

Eisdorfer, E., & Cohen, D. the cognitively impaired elderly: Differential diagnosis. In M. Storandt, I. Siegler & M. Elias, eds., *The clinical psychology of the aging*. New York: Plenum Press, 1978.

Epstein, L. Symposium on age differentiation in depressive illness: Depression in the elderly. *Journal of Gerontology*, 1976, *31*, 278-282.

Erikson, E. H. *Identity and the life cycle*. New York: International Universities Press, 1959.

Erikson, E. H. *Identity: Youth and crisis*. New York: W. W. Norton & Co., 1968.

Falloon, I. R. H. The therapy of depression: A behavioral approach. *Psychotherapy and Psychosomatics*, 1975, *25*, 69-75.

Fann, W. E. Pharmacotherapy in older depressed patients. *Journal of Gerontology*, 1976, *31*, 304-310.

Fann, W. E., & Wheless, J. C. Depression in elderly patients. *Southern Medical Journal*, 1975, *68*, 468-472.

Fassler, L. B., & Gaviria, M. G. Depression in old age. *Journal of the American Geriatrics Society*, 1978, *26*, 471-475.

Feifel, H., & Ellis, J. Patients and therapists assess the same psychotherapy. *Journal of Consulting Psychology*, 1963, *27*, 310-318.

Feigenbaum, E. M. *A geriatric psychiatric outpatient project*. San Francisco: Langley Porter Neuropsychiatric Institute, 1970.

Feigenbaum, E. M. Geriatric psychopathology—internal or external? *Journal of the American Geriatric Society*, 1974, *22*, 49.

Fenichel, O. *The psychoanalytic theory of neurosis*. New York: Norton, 1945.

Fierman, L. B. Myths in the practice of psychotherapy. *Archives of General Psychiatry*, 1965, *12*, 404-414.

Flannery, R. B. Behavior modification of geriatric grief: A transactional perspective. *International Journal of Aging and Human Development*, 1974, *5*, 197-203.

Freud, S. On psychotherapy. *Collected papers.* London: Hogarth Press, 1924.

Friedel, R. O. The pharmacotherapy of depression in the elderly: Pharmacokinetic considerations. In J. O. Cole & J. E. Barrett, eds., *Psychopathology in the aged.* New York: Raven Press, 1980.

Friedman, A. S. Interaction of drug therapy with marital therapy in depressive patients. *Archives of General Psychiatry*, 1975, *32*, 619-637.

Gallagher, D. Behavior group therapy with the elderly. Paper presented at the meeting of the American Psychological Association. New York, August 1979.

Gardner, P., & Oei, T. Depression and self-esteem: An investigation that used behavioral and cognitive approaches to the treatment of clinically depressed clients. *Journal of Clinical Psychology*, 1981, *37*, 128-135.

Garner, H. H., & Korzeniowski, S. The older patient: A confrontation problem-solving technique in treatment. *Postgraduate Medicine*, 1971, *49*, 202-208.

Gauthier, J., & Marshall, W. Grief: A cognitive-behavioral analysis. *Cognitive Therapy and Research*, 1977, *1*, 39-44.

Gendlin, E., & Rychlak, S. Psychotherapeutic processes. *Annual Review of Psychology*, 1970, *21*, 155-190.

Gerner, R. H. Depression in the elderly. In O. Kaplan, ed., *psychopathology of aging.* New York: Academic Press, 1979.

Gilbert, J. G. *Psychotherapy with the aged. Psychotherapy: Theory, Research and Practice*, 1977, *14*, 394-402.

Gitelson, M. The emotional problems of elderly people. *Geriatrics*, 1948, *3*, 135-150.

Gitelson, M. A transference reaction in a sixty-six year old woman. In M. A. Berezin & S. H. Cath eds., *Geriatric Psychiatry*. New York: International Universities Press, 1965.

Glenwick, D. S., & Whitbourne, S. Beyond despair and disengagement: A transactional model of personality development in later life. *International Journal of Aging and Human Development*, 1977, *8*, 261-267.

Godbole, A., & Verinis, J. Brief psychotherapy in the treatment of emotional disorders in physically ill geriatric patients. *Gerontologist*, 1974, *14*, 143-152.

Goldfarb, A. I. Group therapy with the old and aged. In H. I. Kaplan & B. J. Sadock, eds. *Comprehensive group psychotherapy*. Baltimore: Williams & Wilkins, 1971.

Goldfarb, A. I. Minor maladjustments of the aged. In S. Arieti & E. Brody, eds. *American handbook of psychiatry*. New York: Basic Books, 1974.

Goldfarb, A. I. Psychotherapy of aged persons, IV: One aspect of the psychodynamics of the therapeutic situation with aged patients. *Psychoanalytic Review*, 1955, *42*, 180-187.

Goldfarb, A. I. The rationale for psychotherapy with older persons. *American Journal of Medical Science*, 1956, *232*, 181-185.

Goldstein, S. E. Depression in the elderly. *Journal of the American Geriatrics Society*, 1979, *27*, 38-41.

Gottesman, L. E., Quarterman, C. E., & Cohn, G. M. Psychosocial treatment of the aged. In C. Eisdorfer & M. Lawton, eds. *The psychology of adult development and aging*. Washington, D. C.: APA 1973.

Gralewicz, A. Restoration therapy: An approach to group therapy for the chronically ill. *American Journal of Occupational Therapy*, 1968, *22*, 194-199.

Grigorian, H. Aging and depression: The involutional and geriatric patient. In A. J. Enelow, ed. *Depression in medical practice*. West Point: Merck, Sharp & Dohme, 1970.

Grotjahn, M. Analytic therapy with the elderly. *Psychoanalytic Review*, 1955, *42*, 419-427.

Gurland, B. J. The comparative frequency of depression in various adult age groups. *Journal of Gerontology*, 1976, *31*, 283-292.

Hamilton, M. A rating scale for depression. *Journal of Neurology, Neurosurgery and Psychiatry*, 1960, *23*, 56-61.

Hammer, M. Psychotherapy with the aged. In M. Hammer, ed. *The theory and practice of psychotherapy with specific disorders*. Sprinfield, Ill.: Thomas, 1972.

Harris, J. E., & Bodden, J. L. An active group experience for disengaged elderly persons. *Journal of Counseling Psychology*, 1978, *25*, 325-330.

Hartmann, H. *Ego psychology and the problem of adaptation*. New York: International Universities Press, 1958.

Hauser, S. T. The psychotherapy of a depressed aged woman. *Journal of Geriatric Psychiatry*, 1968, *2*.

Havinghurst, R. J. *Human development and education*. New York: David McKay, 1953.

Havinghurst, R. J. Personality and social adjustment in old age. In W. Donahue & C. Tibbitts, ed., *The new frontiers of aging*. Ann Arbor: University of Michigan Press, 1957.

Havinghurst, R. J. Successful aging. In R. H. Williams, C. Tibbitts & W. Donahue, eds., *Processes of aging*. New York: Atherton Press, 1963.

Havinghurst, R. J., & Albrecht, R. *Older people.* New York: Longmans and Green, 1953.

Havinghurst, R. J., Neugarten, B. L., & Tobin, S. S. Disengagement and patterns of aging. Presented at the International Gerontological Research Seminar, Sweden, August 1963.

Havinghurst, R. J., Neugarten, B. L., & Tobin, S. S. Disengagement and patterns of aging. In B. Neugarten, ed. *Middle age and aging: A reader in social psychology.* Chicago: University of Chicago Press, 1968.

Henry, W. E. Engagement and disengagement: Toward a theory of adult development. In R. Kastenbaum, ed., *Contributions to the psychobiology of aging.* New York: Springer, 1965.

Hiatt, H. Dynamic psychotherapy in later life. *Current Psychiatric Therapies,* 1975, *15,* 117-122.

Hiatt, H. Dynamic psychotherapy with the aging patient. *American Journal of Psychotherapy,* 1971, *25,* 591-600.

Howells, J. G. *Principles of family psychiatry.* New York: Brunner/Mazel, 1975.

Hoyer, W. J., Mishara, B. L., & Riedel, R. Problem behaviors as operants. *The Gerontologist,* 1975, *15,* 452-465.

Hussian, R. A., & Lawrence, P. S. Social reinforcement of activity and problem-solving training in the treatment of depressed institutionalized elderly patients. *Cognitive Therapy and Research,* 1981, *5,* 57-69.

Ingebretsen, R. Psychotherapy with the elderly. *Psychotherapy: Theory, Research and Practice,* 1977, *14,* 319-332.

Ingersoll, B., & Silverman, A. Comparative group

psychology for the aged. *The Gerontologist*, 1978, *18*, 201-206.

Jarvik, L. F. Aging and depression: Some unanswered questions. *Journal of Gerontology*, 1976, *31*, 324-326.

Jelliffee, S. E. The old age factor in psychoanalytic therapy. *Medical Journal Record*, 1925, *121*, 7-12.

Jung, C. G., *Psychological reflections: a new anthology of his writings, 1905-1961*. Princeton, N. J.: Bollingen, Princeton University Press, 1972.

Karpf, R. J. Modalities of psychotherapy with the elderly. *Journal of the American Geriatrics Society*, 1980, *28*, 367-371.

Karpf, R. J. The psychotherapy of depression. *Psychotherapy: Theory, Research and Practice*, 1977, *14*, 349-353.

Kastenbaum, R. Personality theory, therapeutic approaches, and the elderly client. In M. Storandt, I. Siegler & M. Elias, eds., *The clinical psychology of aging*. New York: Plenum Press, 1978.

Kaufman, M. R. Old age and aging. *American Journal of Orthopsychiatry*, 1940, *10*, 73-84.

Kaufman, M. R. Psychoanalysis in later life depressions. *Psychoanalytic Quarterly*, 1937, *6*, 308-335.

Kendell, R. E., & Discipio, W. J. Obsessional symptoms and obsessional personality traits in patients with depressive illnesses. *Psychological Medicine*, 1970, *1*, 65-72.

Kivett, V. R., Watson, J. A., & Busch, J. C. The relative importance of physical psychological and social variables to locus of control orientation in middle age. *Journal of Gerontology*, 1977, *32*, 203-210.

Klerman, G. L. Age and clinical depression: Today's youth in the twenty-first century. *Journal of Gerontology*, 1976, *31*, 318-323.

Klerman, G. L. Clinical phenomenology of depression: Implications for research strategy in the psychobiology of the affective disorders. In T. A. Wiliams, M. A. Katz, & J. A. Shields, Jr., eds., *Recent advances in the psychobiology of the depressive illnesses.*

Klerman, G. L., DiMascio, A., Weissman, M. M., Prusoff, B., & Paykel, E. S. Treatment of depression by drugs and psychotherapy. *American Journal of Psychiatry*, 1974, *131*, 186-191.

Knight, B. Psychotherapy and behavior change with the non-institutionalized aged. *International Journal of Aging Human Development*, 1979, *9*, 221-236.

Kovacs, M. M. The efficacy of cognitive and behavior therapies for depression. *American Journal of Psychiatry*, 1980, *137*, 1495-1501.

Kovacs, M. M., Rush, A. J., Beck, A. T., & Hollon, S. I. Depressed outpatients treated with cognitive therapy or pharmacotherapy: A one year follow-up. *Archives of General Psychiatry*, 1981, *38*, 33-39.

Kral, V. A. Somatic therapies in older depressed patients. *Journal of Gerontology*, 1976, *31*, 311-313.

Kramer, C., Kramer, J., & Dunlop, H. Resolving grief. *Geriatric Nursing*, 1966, *2*, 14-17.

Krasner, J. D. Loss of dignity-courtesy of modern science. *Psychotherapy: Theory, Research and Practice*, 1977, *14*, 309-318.

Krasner, L. Behavior therapy. *Annual Review of Psychology*, 1971, *22*, 483-532.

Lago, D., & Hoffman, S. Structured group interaction: An intervention strategy for the continued development of elderly populations. *International Journal of Aging and Human Development*, 1978, *8*, 311-324.

Langley, G. E. Functional psychoses. In J. G. Howells, ed. *Modern perspectives in the psychiatry of old age.* New York: Brunner/Mazel, 1975.

Lazarus, A., & Fay, A. *I can if I want to*. New York: William Morrow, 1975.

Lazarus, L. W. A program for the elderly at a private psychiatric hospital. *Gerontologist*, 1976, *16*, 125--131.

Lefcourt, H. M. The function of the illusions of control and freedom. *American Psychologist*, 1973, *28*, 417-425.

Levin, S. Depression in the aged: A study of the salient external factors. *Geriatrics*, 1963, *18*, 302-307.

Levin, S. Depression in the aged: The importance of external factors. In R. Kastenbaum, ed., *New thoughts on old age*. New York: Springer, 1964.

Levin, S. Depression in the aged. In M. A. Berezin & S. H. Cath, eds., *Geriatric psychiatry*. New York: International Universities Press, 1965.

Levin, S., & Kahana, R. J., eds. *Psychodynamic studies on aging: Creativity, reminiscing and dying*. New York: International Universities Press, 1967.

Levine, B., & Schild, J. Group therapy of depression. *Social Work*, 1969, *14*, 46-52.

Levitt, E. E., & Lublin, B. *Depression*. New York: Springer, 1975.

Levy, S. M., Derogatis, L. R., Gallagher, D., & Gatz, M. Intervention with older adults and the evaluation of outcome. In L. W. Poon, Ed., *Aging in the 1980's*. Washington, D. C.: APA, 1980.

Lewinsohn, P. M. A behavioral approach to depression. In R. J. Friedman & M. M. Katz, eds., *The psychology of depression: Contemporary theory and research*. New York: John Wiley, 1974.

Lewinsohn. P. M. Engagement in pleasant activities and depression level. *Journal of Abnormal Psychology*, 1975, *84*, 729-731.

Lewinsohn, P. M. & Lee, W. L. Assessment of affective

disorders. In D. H. Barlow, ed., *Behavioral assessment of adult disorders*. New York: Guilford Press, 1981.

Lewis, M. I., & Butler, R. N. Life review therapy: Putting memories to work in individual and group psychotherapy. *Geriatrics*, 1974, *29*, 165-173.

Liederman, P., Green, R., & Liederman, V. Outpatient group therapy with geriatric patients. *Geriatrics*, 1967, *22*, 148-153.

Liederman, P., & Liederman, V. Group therapy: An approach to problems of geriatric outpatients. In J. H. Messernan, ed., *Current Psychiatric Therapies*, Vol. 7. New York: Grune & Stratton, 1967.

Linden, M. Group psychotherapy with institutionalized senile women: Studies in gerontologic human relations. *International Journal of Group Psychotherapy*, 1953, *3*, 150-170.

Linn, M. W. Assessing community adjustment in the elderly. In A. Raskin & L. F. Jarvik, eds. *psychiatric symptoms and cognitive loss in the elderly*. New York: John Wiley & Sons, 1979.

Lipman, A., & Smith, K. Functionality of disengagement in old age. *Journal of Gerontology*, 1968, *23*, 517-521.

Lipman, R., & Covi, L. Outpatient treatment of neurotic depression: Medication and group psychotherapy. In R. L. Spitzer & D. F. Klein, eds., *Evaluation of psychological therapies*. Baltimore: Johns Hopkins, 1976.

Lipman, R., Covi, L., & Smith, V. Prediction of response to drug and group psychotherapy in depressed outpatients. *Psychopharmacology Bulletin*, 1975, *11*, Abstract 38.

Lippincott, R. C. Depressive illness: identification and treatment in the elderly. *Geriatrics*, 1968, *23*, 149-152.

Lipton, M. A. Age differentiation in depression: Biochemical aspects. *Journal of Gerontology*, 1976, *31*, 293-299.

Lowenthal, M. F., & Haven, C. Interaction and adaptation: Itinerary as a critical variable. In B. L. Neugarten, ed., *Middle age and aging*. Chicago: University of Chicago Press, 1968.

Lunghi, M. E. The stability of mood and social perception measures in a sample of depressive inpatients. *British Journal of Psychiatry*, 1977, *130*, 598-604.

Maddox, G. L. Sociological perspectives in gerontological research. In D. Kent, R. Kastenbaum, & S. Sherwood, eds. *Research planning and action for the elderly*. New York: Behavioral Publications, 1972.

Maier, S. F., & Seligman, M. E. Learned helplessness: Theory and evidence. *Journal of Experimental Psychology*, 1976, *105*, 3-46.

Mardoyan, J. L., Weis, D. M. The efficacy of group counseling with older adults. *Personnel and Guidance Journal*, 1981, 161-163.

Meerloo, J. A. Modes of psychotherapy in the aged. *Journal of the American Geriatric Society*, 1961, *9*, 225-234.

Meerloo, J. A. Transference and resistance in geriatric psychotherapy. *Psychoanalytic Review*, 1955, *42*, 78-82.

Mintz, J., Steuer, J., & Jarvik, L. Psychotherapy with depressed elderly patients: Research considerations. *Journal of Consulting and Clinical Psychology*, 1981, *49*, 542-548.

Moss, R. E. Aging: A survey of the psychiatric literature. In M. A. Berezin & S. H. Cath, eds., *Geriatric psychiatry: Grief, loss and emotional disorders in the aging process*. New York: International Universities Press, 1965.

Nehrke, M. F., Hulicka, I. M., & Morganit, J. E. Age differences in life satisfaction, locus of control, and self concept. *International Journal of Aging and Human Development*, 1980, *11*, 25-33.

Neiderehe, G. Paper presented at 30th annual scientific meeting of the Gerontological Society, San Francisco, November 20, 1977.

Neugarten, B. L. *Middle age and aging*. Chicago: University of Chicago Press, 1968.

Neugarten, B. L. Personality change in late life: A developmental perspective. In C. Eisdorfer & M. P. Lawton, eds., *The psychology of adult development and aging*. Washington, D. C.: American Psychiatric Association, 1973.

Neumann, C. P. Depression in the aged: Its diagnosis and treatment. *Connecticut Medicine*, 1974, *38*, 403.

Nowlin, J. B., & Busse, E. W. Psychosomatic problems in the older person. In E. D. Witkower & H. Warnes, eds., *Psychosomatic medicine*. New York: Harper and Row, 1977.

Oberleder, M. Crisis therapy in mental breakdown of the aging. *Gerontologist*, 1970, *10*, 111-114.

O'Brien, C. R., Johnson, J. L., & Miller, B. Counseling the aging: Some practical considerations. *Personnel & Guidance Journal*, 1979, *57*, 288-291.

Ohlsen, M. M. *Group Counseling*. New York: Holt, Rinehart & Winston, 1977.

Oradei, D., & Waite, N. Group psychotherapy with stroke patients during the immediate recovery phase. *American Journal of Orthopsychiatry*, 1974, *44*, 386-395.

Palmore, E. B. The effects of aging on activities and attitudes. *Gerontologist*, 1968, *8*, 259-263.

Palmore, E. B. Social factors in mental illness of the aged. In E. W. Busse & E. Pfeiffer, eds., *Mental illness in later life*. Washington, D. C.: American Psychiatric Association, 1973.

Palmore, E. B., & Luikart, C. Health and social factors related to life satisfaction. *Journal of Health and Social Behavior*, 1972, *13*, 68-80.

Pappas, M., Page, C., & Baker, J. A controlled study of an intensive treatment program for hospitalized geriatric patients. *Journal of the American Geriatrics Society*, 1958, *6*, 17-26.

Paykel, E. S., Myers, J. K., Dienelt, M. N., Klerman, G. L., Lindenthal, J. J., & Pepper, M. P. Life events and depression. *Archives of General Psychiatry*, 1969, *21*, 735-760.

Peck, A. Psychotherapy of the aged. *Journal of the American Geriatrics Society*, 1966, *14*, 748-753.

Peterson, J. A. Marital and family therapy involving the aged. *Gerontologist*, 1973, *13*, 27-31.

Petty, B., Moeller, T., & Campbell, R. Support groups for elderly persons in the community. *Gerontologist*, 1976, *16*, 522-529.

Pfeiffer, E. Psychotherapy with elderly patients. *Postgraduate Medicine*, 1971, *50*, 254-258.

Pfeiffer, E., & Busse, E. W. Mental disorders in later life: Affective disorders; paranoid, neurotic, and situational reactions. In E. W. Busse & E. Pfeiffer, eds., *Mental illness in later life*. Washington, D. C.: American Psychiatric Association, 1973.

Phillips, J. S., & Bierman, K. L. Clinical psychology: Individual methods. *Annual Review of Psychology*, 1981, 405-438.

Pincus, A. Reminiscence in aging and its implications for social work practice. *Social Work*, 1970, *15*, 47-53.

Pitt, B. *Psychogeriatrics*. London: Churchill Livingstone, 1974.

Portnoi, V. A., & Shriber, L. S. Management of the

mental health of ambulatory elderly patients. *Journal of the American Geriatrics Society*, 1980, *38*, 325-330.

Radebold, H. Psychoanalytic group psychotherapy with older adults: Report on specific issues. *Zeitschrift fur Gerontologie*, 1976, *9*, 128-142.

Raskin, A. Signs and symptoms of psychopathology in the elderly. In A. Raskin & L. Jarvik, eds., *Psychiatric symptoms and cognitive loss in the elderly*. Washington: Hemisphere, 1979.

Raskind, M., & Eisdorfer, C. Psychopharmacology in the aged. In L. L. Simpson, ed., *Drug treatment of mental disorders*. New York: Raven Press, 1976.

Rechtschaffen, A. Intensive treatment program for state geriatric patients. *Geriatrics*, 1954, *9*, 28-34.

Rechtschaffen, A. Psychotherapy with geriatric patients: A review of the literature. *Gerontology*, 1959, *14*, 73-84.

Reid, D. W., Haas, G., & Hawkings, D. Locus of desired control and positive self-concept of the elderly. *Journal of Gerontology*, 1977, *32*, 441-450.

Richards, W. S., & Thorpe, G. L. Behavioral approaches to the problems of later life. In M. Storandt, J. Siegler & M. Elias, eds., *The clinical psychology of aging*. New York: Plenum Press, 1978.

Riedel, R. G. Experimental analysis as applied to adulthood and old age: A review. A paper presented at the meeting of the American Psychological Association, New Orleans, August, 1974.

Rockwell, F. V. Psychotherapy and the older individual. In O. J. Kaplan, ed., *Mental disorders of later life*. Stanford: Stanford University Press, 1956.

Rose, A. A current theoretical issue in social gerontology. *Gerontologist*, 1964, *4*, 46-50.

Rosenbaum, J., Friedlander, J., & Kaplan, S. Evaluation of results of psychotherapy. *Psychosomatic*

Medicine, 1956, *18*, 113-132.

Rosenthal, H. R. Psychotherapy of the aging. *American Journal of Psychotherapy*, 1959, *13*, 55-65.

Roth, M. The natural history of mental disorders in old age. *Journal of Mental Science*, 1955, *101*, 281-301.

Rotter, J. B. Generalized expectancies for internal versus external control of reinforcement. *Psychological Monographs*, 1966, *80*, 609.

Rounsaville, B. J., Klerman, G. L., & Weissman, M. M. Do psychotherapy and pharmocotherapy for depression conflict? *Archives of General Psychiatry*, 1981, *38*, 24-29.

Rounsaville, B. J., Weissman, M. M., & Prusoff, B. A. Psychotherapy with depressed outpatients: Patient and process variables as predictors of outcome. *British Journal of Psychiatry*, 1981, *138*, 67-74

Rush, A. J., Beck, A. T., Kovacs, M., & Hollon, S. I. Comparative efficacy of cognitive therapy and pharmocotherapy in the treatment of depressed outpatients. *Cognitive Therapy Research*, 1977, *1*, 17-37.

Safirstein, S. L. Psychotherapy for geriatric patients. *New York State Journal of Medicine*, 1972, *72*, 2743-2748.

Salzman, C., & Shader, R. I. Clinical evaluation of depression in the elderly. In A. Raskin & L. F. Jarvik, eds. *Psychiatric symptoms and cognitive loss in the elderly*. Washington, D. C.: Hemisphere, 1979.

Salzman, C., & Shader, R. I. Depression in the elderly. I. Relationship between depression, psychologic defense mechanisms and physical illness. *Journal of the American Geriatrics Society*, 1978, *26*, 253-259.

Salzman, C., & Shader, R. I. Depression in the elderly, II. Possible drug etiologies; differential diagnostic criteria. *Journal of the American Geriatrics Society*, 1978, *26*, 303-308.

Schmidt, C. W., Jr. Psychiatric problems of the aged.

Journal of the American Geriatrics Society, 1974, *22*, 355-359.

Scott, J., & Gaitz, C. M. Ethnic and age difference in mental health measurements. *Diseases of the Nervous System*, 1975, *36*, 389-393.

Seegal, D. Principles of geriatric care. *Journal of Chronic Diseases*, 1956, *3*, 100-103.

Seeman, J. Counselor judgements of therapeutic process and outcome. In C. R. Rodgers & R. F. Dymond, eds., *Psychotherapy and personality change.* Chicago: University of Chicago Press, 1954.

Segal, H. Fear of death: Notes on the analysis of an old man. *International Journal of Psychoanalysis*, 1958, *39*, 178-181.

Seligman, M. E. Comment and integrations. *Journal of Abnormal Psychology*, 1978, *87*, 165-179.

Seligman, M. E. *Helplessness.* San Francisco: Freeman, 1975.

Shaw, B. F. Comparison of cognitive therapy and behavior therapy in the treatment of depression. *Journal of Consulting and Clinical Psychology*, 1977, *45*, 543-551.

Silver, A. Group psychotherapy with senile psychotic patients. *Geriatrics*, 1950, *5*, 147-150.

Smith, M. Sociometic changes in a group of adult female psychotics following an intensive socializing program. *Group Psychotherapy*, 1951, *4*, 145-155.

Solomon, K. The depressed patient: Social antecedents of psychopathologic changes in the elderly. *Journal of the American Geriatrics Society*, 1981, *29*, 14-18.

Sparacino, J. Individual psychotherapy with the aged: A review. *International Journal of Aging and Human Development*, 1979, *9*, 197-220.

Spicer, C. C., Hare, H., & Slater, E. neurotic and psychotic forms of depressive illness: Evidence from age-incidence in a national sample. *British Journal of Psychiatry*, 1973, *123*, 535-541.

Stonecypher, D. D. *Growing older and staying younger.* New York: Norton, 1974.

Storandt, M. Other approaches to therapy. In M. Storandt, I. Seigler & M. Elias, eds., *The clinical psychology of aging.* New York: Plenum Press, 1978.

Strickland, B. R. Locus of control: Where have we been and where are we going? Paper presented at American Psychological Association meeting, Montreal, 1973.

Swab, J. J., Holzer, C. E., & Warheti, G. J. Depressive symptomology and age. *Psychosomatics*, 1973, *14*, 135-141.

Verwoerdt, A. *Clinical geropsychiatry.* Baltimore: Williams & Wilkins, 1976.

Vickers, R. The therapeutic milieu and the older depressed patient. *Journal of Gerontology*, 1976, *31*, 314-317.

Wasser, E. *Creative approaches in casework with the aging.* New York: Family Service Association of America, 1966.

Waters, E., Fink, S., & White, B. Peer group counseling for older people. *Educational Gerontology*, 1976, *1*, 157-169.

Wayne, G. J. Psychotherapy in senescence. *Annals of Western Medicine and Surgery*, 1952, *6*, 88-91.

Wayne, G. J. Modified psychoanalytic therapy in senescence. *Psychoanalytic Review*, 1953, *40*, 99-116.

Weinberg, J. Psychiatric techniques in the treatment of older people. In W. Donahue & C. Tibbitts, eds., *Growing in the older years.* Ann Arbor: University of Michigan Press, 1951.

Weinberg, J. Psychopathology. In J. G. Howells, ed., *Modern perspectives in the psychiatry of old age.* New York: Brunner/Mazel, 1975.

Weinberg, J. Psychotherapy of the aged. In J. H. Masserman, & J. L. Moreno, eds., *Progress in psychotherapy, anxiety and therapy.* New York: Grune & Stratton, 1957, Vol. 2.

Weinberg, J. Psychotherapy of the aged gratifies, challenges the therapist. *Frontiers of Clinical Psychiatry* (Roche Laboratories), 1970, *5.*

Weiss, J. A. Suicide. In S. Arieti & E. Brody, eds., *American handbook of psychiatry*, Vol. 3., Second Edition. New York: Basic Books, 1974.

Weissman, M. Psychotherapy and its relevance to the pharmacology of affective disorders: From ideology to evidence. In M. A. Lipton, A. DiMascio & K. F. Killam, eds., *Psychopharmacology: A generation of progress.* New York: Raven Press, 1978.

Weissman, M., Klerman, G., Paykel, E., Prusoff, B., & Hanson, B. Treatment effects on the social adjustment of depressed patients. *Archives of General Psychiatry*, 1974, *31*, 771-778.

Weissman, M., Prusoff, B., DiMascio, A., Neu, C., Goklaney, M., & Klerman, G. The efficacy of drugs and psychotherapy in the treatment of acute depressive episodes. *American Journal of Psychiatry*, 1979, *136*, 555-558.

White, R. W. *Ego and reality.* New York: International Universities Press, 1963.

Whitehead, J. M. *Psychiatric disorders in old age.* New York: Springer, 1974.

Wilensky, H., & Weiner, M. B. Facing reality in psycotherapy with the aging. *Psychotherapy: Theory, Research and Practice*, 1977, *14*, 373-377.

Willner, M. Individual psychotherapy with the

depressed elderly outpatient: An overview. *Journal of the American Geriatrics Society,* 1978, *26*, 231-235.

Wolberg, L. R. Resistance to cure in psychotherapy. *New York State Journal of Medicine,* 1943b, *43*, 1751-1754.

Wolff, K. *The emotional rehabilitation of the geriatric patient.* Springfield, Ill.: Thomas, 1970.

Wolff, K. *Geriatric psychiatry.* Springfield, Ill.: Thomas, 1963.

Wolff, K. Group psychotherapy with geriatric patients in a mental hospital. *Journal of the American Geriatrics Society,* 1957, *5*, 13-19.

Wolff, K. Individual psychotherapy with geriatric patients. *Psychosomatics,* 1971, *12*, 89-94.

Wolff, K. The treatment of the depressed and suicidal geriatric patient. *Geriatrics,* 1971, 65-69.

Wolff, K. Treatment of the geriatric patient in a mental hospital. *Journal of the American Geriatrics Society,* 1956, *4*, 472-476.

Wolk, S. Situational constraint as a moderator of the locus of control-adjustment relationship. *Journal of Consulting and Clinical Psychology,* 1976, *44*, 420-427.

Wolk, S., & Kurtz, J. Positive adjustment and involvement during aging and expectancy for internal control. *Journal of Consulting and Clinical Psychology,* 1975, *43*, 173-178.

Wong, P.T.P., & Sproule, C.F. An attribution analysis of the locus of control construct and the Trent attribution profile. In Herbert M. Lefcourt ed., *Research with the locus of control construct,* Vol. 3. Extensions and limitations. New York: Academic Press, 1984.

Woodruff, R. A., Goodwin, D. W., & Guze, S. B. *Psychiatric diagnosis.* New York: Oxford, 1974.

Zarsky, E. L., & Blau, D. The understanding and management of narcissistic regression and dependency in an elderly woman observed over an extended period of time. *Journal of Geriatric Psychiatry*, 1970, *3*, 160.

Zinberg, N. E. Geriatric psychiatry: Needs and problems. *Gerontologist*, 1967, *4*, 130-135.

Zinberg, N. E. & Kaufman, I. Cultural and personality factors associated with aging: An introduction. In N. Zinberg, ed., *The normal psychology of the aging process*. New York: International Universities Press, 1963.

GLOSSARY

Acute psychotic depression: a sudden onset of severe depressive mood which may block awareness of reality.

Affective disorders: disturbance of mood accompanied by a full or partial manic or depressive syndrome that is not due to any other physical or mental disorder.

Analytic-dynamic: a term used to describe a number of the classic theoretical systems of psychology and psychotherapy that view unconscious processes as prime motivators and determinants of behaviors.

Bipolar depression: an affective disorder characterized by chronic depressed mood with at least one episode of excessive elation or agitation.

Cerebral arteriosclerosis: hardening of the arteries in the brain; sometimes results in an organic brain syndrome that may be neurological and/or psychological in nature.

Change score: a score derived from a comparison of an individual's current level of performance on a particular measure against a prior level of performance on that measure.

Chronic brain dysfunction: a long-term, generally

169

irreversible change or disturbance in the function of the brain and central nervous system, usually characterized by impairments in one or more of the following areas: basic arousal and orientation, intellectual processes, abstract reasoning, memory. Also may be accompanied by or preceded by changes in mood and personality organization. *See also* Senile dementia.

Clinical depression: a disorder in which there are depressive symptoms that meet the criteria for a formal diagnosis—as opposed to a sad mood resulting from everyday "blues."

Cognitive behavioral therapy: a problem-focused therapeutic approach that emphasizes the role of feelings, thoughts and other covert mental processes in mediating emotional dysfunction.

Confound: a situation in an experiment in which unambiguous interpretation of results is rendered impossible, either because the design of the experiment is poor, or because other unforeseen factors not directly under the control of the experimenter are directly affecting the outcome.

Contingent social reinforcement: social rewards (i.e., attention, smiles, head nods) given to an individual only upon the emission of a particular desired behavior.

Contracting: a simple therapeutic strategy in which a formal or informal agreement, with specified objectives, outcomes and consequences, is negotiated between the patient and therapist.

Dependent measure: any measurement of an individual's performance after exposure to an experimental condition or manipulation. The manipulations of an experiment themselves are said to be the independent variables.

Developmental tasks: age-appropriate skills or abilities related to emotional and/ or physical functioning of the individual.

Differential diagnosis: the process of identifying a specific mental or physical disorder as the one most likely to be the cause of the individual's illness.

Differential reinforcement values: different levels of response from individuals who have been given the same rewards.

Differential treatment responses: individual and/or group differences in level and degree of response to a particular experimental manipulation.

Ego-dystonic symptoms: personality traits recognized by the individual as unacceptable and undesirable.

Ego-syntonic symptoms: traits recognized by the individual as acceptable and non-distressing.

Electroconvulsive therapy: use of electric current to induce unconsciousness and/or convulsive seizures; mostly used in treatment of severe depression.

Endogenous psychotic depression: *See* psychotic-endogenous depression.

Hypochondriasis: a condition characterized by persistent preoccupation with physical health.

Imagal exposure: exposure to images. In this case, presentation of photographs of deceased loved ones to patients in order to elicit and ultimately extinguish depressive affect associated with memories of the deceased.

Insight-analytic therapy: *See* insight-oriented dynamic therapy.

Insight-oriented dynamic therapy: method of psychotherapy based on the belief that psychological health is best promoted by an exploration and understanding of the largely unconscious roots of maladaptive behavior or emotional conflict. The primary objective of such therapy is the facilitation of conscious awareness and understanding of the mechanisms of emotional conflict. This understanding is essential if change in personality and behavior is to occur.

Intrapsychic defenses: unconscious processes used to relieve anxieties and conflicts that arise from one's own impulses and drives.

Life review technique: a structured therapeutic approach using reminiscence to help older persons constructively evaluate past accomplishments and become aware of inherenct capabilities and limitations for coping with the aging process.

Milieu therapy: an approach in which all interpersonal relations in the individual's environment are viewed as potentially therapeutic. Major emphasis is placed upon active development of social skills.

Neurotic-reactive depression: a type of depression assumed to be influenced by everyday environmental stressors such as loss of job, illness or marital problems.

Operant methods: use of rewarding and/or punishing consequences to either increase or decrease the frequency of a selected behavior.

Parsimonious: in the sciences, refers to the most concise interpretation possible for a given occurrence, event, or phenomenon.

Premorbid personality: an individual's characteristic set of behavior patterns including physical and mental activities, attitudes and interests, prior to the onset of emotional disorder.

Problem-solving coping skills therapy: type of behavioral therapy in which there is a structured approach to defining and solving life-problems; a problem is broken down into various components, each with its own specified goal or outcome. This often involves helping the individual to learn new ways of adjusting to environmental stress without altering essential goals or objectives.

Psychomotor retardation: visible generalized slowing down of physical reactions, movements and speech.

Psychotic-endogenous depression: a more severe form of depression believed to be biochemical in origin. Symptoms respond more favorably to psychopharmacological treatment interventions coupled with a secondary emphasis on improving one's adaptation to the environment.

Reality therapy: a structured technique used to assist individuals who are experiencing disorientation. Attemtps are made to enable them to become more self-sufficient and more interested in and aware of people and events in their environment.

Resocialization therapy: a structured group program for geriatric patients. Stress is on improving interpersonal relations and helping the individual establish renewed interest in the environment through activities designed to enhance social behaviors.

Rorschach: a projective measure of personality using a patient's associations in response to a series of inkblots.

Self-statements: covert thoughts expressed by an individual about him or herself that may be influencing self-perception, attitudes and behavior.

Senile dementia: loss of intellectual abilities of sufficient severity to interfere with social or occupation functioning; changes in personality and behavior also occur. Symptoms may vary in severity but the course is generally progressive.

Somatization: expression of a psychological problem primarily in terms of physical symptoms.

Thematic Apperception Test: a projective instrument.

that requires the individual to compose stories based on the viewing of stimulus pictures.

Unipolar depression: affective disorder characterized by chronic and recurring depressive mood state.

Weschler-Bellevue Intelligence Scale: original form of the Weschler Adult Intelligence Scale, published in 1939. It consists of a variety of subtests assessing both verbal and nonverbal performance abilities of adults.

NAME INDEX

SUBJECT INDEX

Abandonment, 125
Activity levels, Control group
with high a.l., 130-131;
Higher with internal **Locus
of control**, 52; Increase as
a goal of therapy, 75-76, 83,
97, 130; Increased by **Group
therapy**, 120, 130; Reduced
with external **Locus of
control**, 55, 95; Related to
Depression, 55, 110; Self-
monitoring of, 129; Social,
116, 120
Activity theory, 41, 43-44, 130
Acute Depression, 25, 169; *See
Also* **Psychotic depression**

Adaptation, 4, 29, 30, 33, 35, 83;
Crises in, 35; **Dependency**
as, 92; **Depression as**
normal a. to aging, 135;
Disengagement as index
of, 45; **Loss** as factor in, 38,
39; Poor a. correlated with
Rigidity, 49, 50, 138; Previous to therapy, 74; Promoted in **Group therapy**,
116; Similarity of a. across
the life span, 34, 44; Successful a. of elderly, 32, 44,
83, 85, 86, 88, 130, 138;
Unsuccessful a. related to
Depression, 84; *See also*